ADHD Unpacked

ADHD in Children, Men, and Women—Do I Have ADHD?

Dr. Hong Ji (Doyle) Pi

Table of Contents

Introduction

Megan was a fairly good student in primary school. Her grades were by no means the best in the class, but she was above average. She was also liked by her peers and her teachers and never elicited any behavioral concerns. However, when she was in high school, she started noticing struggles in both her academics and her relationships with her friends.

Friendships weren't the only aspect of her life that she struggled to maintain. Megan also found it difficult to submit assignments on time, remember homework, and study for long periods of time. While she was fully capable of sitting still, she constantly found herself zoning out of having other random thoughts in her mind. One moment, she's learning that the microconidia are the powerhouse of the cell, and the next, she's thinking of that hilarious television program she watched three years ago, wondering if it's still showing.

She battled through high school in silence. Despite her struggles, she often felt that she just needed to try harder. She concealed her struggles to not feel different from her peers. She simply thought she wasn't as smart or likable as some of the other girls in her class. By the time she got to college, she was overwhelmed with stress, which impacted her productivity and mood. Eventually, she sought professional help and received treatment for anxiety and depression. However, even though she saw limited progress, she continued to persevere and hoped that, with time, everything would sort itself out.

After college, Megan entered the workforce, met her husband, and became a mom of two. Despite having a supportive family life, her struggles persevered. It felt like she was running through a rainstorm while trying to stop the droplets from falling to the ground, holding a bucket filled with holes. It felt impossible to remember all the deadlines, pay attention to everyone's needs, get things done at work, be productive, be present, and have any energy remaining to focus on her own passions as well. One day, as she was making school lunches and listening to a podcast, she heard something that changed her life forever. The guest on the podcast was talking about her experience with ADHD, and Megan identified it as a replica of her own life.

Immediately, all Megan could focus on was learning more about ADHD. What she once thought was a disorder that meant you couldn't keep your feet still turned out to be so much more. After learning more about ADHD and seeking professional care, she was diagnosed with ADHD at the age of 34. "But isn't it too late for me?" she asked her doctor. "No, it's never too late. What's important is what you can do moving forward."

Perhaps you feel like Megan—misunderstood, confused, suffering in silence. Or maybe you've had ADHD since you were a toddler. Either way, this book is for you if you're looking to understand ADHD beyond the surface, learn how it can manifest differently in various people, and help find ways to effectively manage your symptoms. Who is this book not for? For anyone looking for a quick fix. I'm sorry to break it to you. ADHD doesn't work that way. In fact, ADHD isn't something you can "cure." However, with the right tools and fundamental truths, you can learn how to manage your ADHD, allowing you to live a more effective, productive, and positive life.

As a psychiatrist, I've seen it happen in so many people: they suffer for years, either trying to get the right diagnosis or trying to manage their ADHD with methods that weren't created for the neurodivergent mind. That's why I've devoted my career to helping individuals with mental health struggles, particularly those with ADHD. I work with my clients, respecting that everyone is unique and no experience is the same. I use a comprehensive approach to understanding each individual's personal needs. Through my work, I've helped many who have been misdiagnosed, as well as those who struggle to understand ADHD and the misconceptions regarding it.

My goal for this book is to advocate for, educate, support, and encourage ADHDers. I want to demystify ADHD while shedding light on how it might manifest uniquely in different people. Don't worry—I'm not writing this book to serve as a textbook. I'll break down complex concepts into digestible bites to make it an easy and enjoyable read, empowering you to improve your mental and physical well-being.

I put a lot of emphasis on the difference in how ADHD manifests in men, women, children, and adults. Why? Because I've seen too many Megans going through life carrying the idea that they aren't good enough because of the way their mind works. Most people would've overlooked Megan's symptoms because they might not look like typical ADHD, but "typical" ADHD is a myth. There were many signs in Megan's life that pointed to ADHD. She actually showed various traits that are typical of ADHD in women—people just weren't aware of it.

In this book, we'll explore what ADHD really is and what it isn't. We'll look at what it might look like in different individuals and how it can impact people in different ways. We'll also explore how ADHD often overlaps with other mental health conditions and why it's important to be aware of it. Later, we'll discover ADHD management strategies that actually work for children and other strategies that will aid management for adults. Lastly, we'll also discuss possible treatment options for ADHD, exploring every possible angle and step of the process.

So, are you ready to have your "ah-ha" moment, just like Megan? Or perhaps you've already had that moment and are now looking for additional knowledge or practical steps? Then you're in the right place, too. Get ready to learn, grow, and gain the knowledge and practical tools you've been waiting for. If you feel overwhelmed or you start getting distracted at any point during this book, don't be too hard on yourself. Take a break, but put a reminder on your phone to get back to reading (before the book ends up underneath a laundry pile, never to be seen again). With that being said, let's not waste another second and jump right in!

Chapter 1:

What is ADHD Really?

We are all a little weird, and life's a little weird, and when we find someone whose weirdness is compatible with ours, we join up with them, fall in mutual weirdness, and call it love. -Dr. Seuss

Often, when someone or their child gets diagnosed with ADHD, the response from family and friends can be mixed. While some are encouraging and uplifting, others stigmatize it. Others simply believe there is no such thing as ADHD and write it off as normal, being naughty, bad parenting, or a poor diet (too much sugar). There are so many misconceptions about ADHD that it makes it difficult for people to really understand what it is and have compassion toward ADHDers.

It's crucial to understand ADHD for yourself before you can expect others to let go of their misconceptions and stereotypes. Consider every piece of unsolicited advice or snarky remark as a sign of a lack of understanding and knowledge. You can only provide insight to people around you if you already understand what it truly is. That's why that's the first place to start on this journey. Before we can look at different treatment options or management techniques, we'll focus on what ADHD truly is— exactly what this chapter aims to do.

The Scientific Breakdown of ADHD

Attention-deficit/hyperactivity disorder (ADHD) is one of the most common and most studied neurodevelopmental disorders (Cleveland Clinic, 2023a). It's a neurological condition that causes executive dysfunction, meaning it disrupts your ability to manage your emotions, thoughts, and actions effectively. Despite a common understanding of how ADHD presents, individuals can unfortunately have either distinctive or atypical presentations.

Types of ADHD

Understanding that there are different types of ADHD is vital if you want to ensure an accurate diagnosis. Recognizing specific ADHD symptoms allows for a more accurate diagnosis, which ensures that individuals receive the appropriate support and treatment. Understanding the different types also reduces the stigmas and dispels misconceptions regarding ADHD. In other words, by being aware of the different types of ADHD, people like Megan are more likely to receive the help they need at a much younger age. ADHD has three distinct subtypes: inattentive, hyperactive-impulsive, and combination.

Inattentive ADHD

Inattentive ADHD is a subtype of ADHD that primarily affects a person's ability to pay attention and focus. It is characterized by difficulties with sustained attention, organization, and task completion. Individuals with this presentation may appear daydreamy, easily distracted, and forgetful. They may struggle to follow instructions, lose things frequently, and have difficulty completing tasks (Cleveland Clinic, 2024b). This type is often less obvious than other types of ADHD, and it can be challenging to diagnose, especially in adults. Symptoms of inattentive ADHD include:

- difficulty paying attention to details and making careless mistakes

- difficulty sustaining attention in tasks or play activities

- difficulty listening when spoken to directly
- difficulty following through on instructions and failing to finish schoolwork, chores, or duties in the workplace (not due to defiance or failure to understand instructions)
- difficulty organizing tasks and activities
- getting easily overwhelmed with tasks
- avoidance of, dislike of, or reluctance to engage in tasks that require sustained mental effort
- losing things necessary for tasks or activities
- easily distracted by extraneous stimuli
- forgetfulness in daily activities

A great example of this is the frustration a client recently shared with me. "My husband would ask me to fetch him something from the bedroom, so I'll start walking toward the bedroom, but halfway down the hallway, I'll forget what I'm doing and yell, 'What do you need again?' He'll answer that he's looking for something specific on his bedside table. So, I'll walk into the bedroom and forget what I'm doing here. 'What are you looking for from the room?' I'll again. 'The flashlight!' I'll walk over to the bedside table where I know he keeps the flashlight, but then I'll forget what he's looking for on his bedside table. 'The flashlight, please!' he'd yell down the hallway before I could ask again. Finally, I'll grab the flashlight, feeling like an absolute failure."

Inattentive ADHD symptoms might be less obvious at first, but that doesn't mean they don't impact a person's daily life. In fact, it can greatly affect academic performance, work productivity, and relationship success (sounds familiar?). For example, a student with inattentive ADHD may have difficulty paying attention in class, leading to poor grades and frustration. An adult with inattentive ADHD may struggle to complete tasks at work, leading to missed deadlines and job dissatisfaction.

Not everyone with inattentive type ADHD will experience all of these symptoms mentioned. ADHD can look different in every person. Therefore, even if some of these symptoms are present and disrupt your everyday life, it's worth investigating.

Hyperactive-Impulsive ADHD

Hyperactive-impulsive ADHD is a subtype of ADHD characterized by symptoms of excessive motor activity, difficulty remaining seated, and impulsive behavior (Cleveland Clinic, 2023a). This type is often more easily recognized, especially in children, since they are often disruptive to others. Hyperactive-impulsive presentation is viewed as the "stereotypical" ADHD. It's the ADHD we often see represented in the media (often inaccurately portrayed), and it's also the type of ADHD that gets diagnosed the fastest. Individuals with this type of ADHD may exhibit the following behaviors:

- fidgeting and squirming in their seats
- running about or climbing excessively
- difficulty engaging in quiet activities
- being "on the go" or driven by a motor
- blurting out answers or interrupting conversations
- difficulty waiting their turn
- engaging in risky or dangerous behaviors without considering the consequences

I recently had a parent describe her son's behavior to me, and without realizing it, she ticked almost all of the hyperactive-impulsive ADHD symptoms. She thought there was something "wrong" with him because he was "acting out." She described him as follows: "He's always busy. He can't just sit down and spend time with us; it is almost like he's hiding something. He won't let me finish speaking, even when I'm expressing concern for his health. He's been in the hospital three times in the last year due to injuries obtained from reckless behavior. He is acting like a squirrel, jumping between tasks without taking a second to breathe." While the mother's concerns were all valid, she had a good kid who was "acting out" because that was the only way he knew how to manage his ADHD symptoms.

It's important to note that the symptoms of hyperactive-impulsive ADHD can vary widely from person to person, and the specific presentation of the disorder can change over time. Even if you never "acted out," it doesn't mean you don't have this type of ADHD. Perhaps you managed your restlessness by participating in every sport your school offered or by going to the bathroom during a meeting even if you didn't have to just get a break.

Combined ADHD

A combined type is exactly what it sounds like: a combination of inattentive and hyperactive-impulsive types. This means you present symptoms from both types of ADHD, not just one (Cleveland Clinic, 2023a). This makes it especially challenging as you'll have to adopt management techniques that work for both types of ADHD.

This is one of the most common neurodevelopmental disorders among children. It's estimated that it affects between five to eight percent of children worldwide (Staley et al., 2024). That percentage drops in adulthood, not because ADHD goes away, but because many adults go without ever getting diagnosed. Even though hyperactive-impulsive ADHD is viewed as the stereotypical type of ADHD, it is not the most prevalent. The most common type of ADHD is the combined type, then inattentive, followed by hyperactive-impulsive (Wilens et al., 2009). The cause of ADHD is unclear, but there are three main ways in which the ADHD brain is different from neurotypical brains. Let's have a closer look.

The Difference Between an ADHD Brain and a Neurotypical Brain

The human brain is a complex and fascinating organ. While most brains function similarly, there are variations in how they are wired and process information. One such variation is observed in individuals with ADHD. While a neurotypical brain, or a brain without ADHD, functions in a way that allows for focused attention, sustained effort, and controlled impulses, an ADHD brain operates differently. The key difference between an ADHD brain and a neurotypical brain lies in three areas: structural difference, chemical signals, and executive function (Cronkleton, 2021).

Structural Differences

Research suggests that ADHDers have different brain structures compared to those without the condition (Wilkins, 2024). These differences often involve areas of the brain responsible for attention, motivation, and behavior regulation, such as the prefrontal cortex, basal ganglia, and cerebellum. Studies have found that in ADHD children, the prefrontal cortex takes longer to mature and is, therefore, also slightly smaller. Similarly, the hippocampus, amygdala, and cerebellum are also smaller in volume within the ADHD mind.

This is important to note because the cerebellum regulates movement. In other words, because of the smaller cerebellum, ADHDers will have trouble sitting still while busy with another task. Additionally, a small hippocampus is connected to poor working memory, emotional regulation issues, and impulsive behavior (Wilkins, 2024).

Chemical Signals

Neurotransmitters are chemical messengers that transmit signals between neurons, and they play a crucial role in brain function. Research suggests that imbalances in certain neurotransmitters, such as dopamine and norepinephrine, may contribute to emotional dysregulation and other ADHD symptoms. Dopamine specifically is involved in motivation, reward, and attention (Silva, 2024). It plays a major role in the brain's reward system, driving individuals to seek out and engage in pleasurable activities. In the context of ADHD, dopamine dysfunction can manifest as:

- **Reduced motivation:** Individuals may experience decreased motivation and difficulty finding activities rewarding, leading to procrastination and difficulty initiating tasks.

- **Difficulty with attention and focus:** Dopamine is essential for maintaining sustained attention and filtering out distractions. Imbalances can lead to difficulties concentrating, easily getting sidetracked, and struggling to complete tasks.

- **Increased impulsivity:** Dopamine also plays a role in impulse control. Dysregulation can contribute to impulsive behaviors, such as interrupting others, acting without thinking, and difficulty waiting for their turn.

Another neurotransmitter that plays a large role in ADHD is norepinephrine. This neurotransmitter is primarily involved in arousal, alertness, and focus. It helps to regulate attention, increase vigilance, and improve cognitive performance (Vanicek et al., 2014). In ADHD, norepinephrine dysfunction can result in:

- **Inattention and distractibility:** Reduced levels of norepinephrine can impair the ability to focus and maintain attention, making it difficult to concentrate on tasks and filter out distractions.

- **Fatigue and difficulty with arousal:** Norepinephrine plays a key role in regulating arousal levels. Imbalances can lead to feelings of fatigue, difficulty waking up, and challenges initiating and sustaining activity.

- **Emotional dysregulation:** Norepinephrine also plays a role in mood regulation. Imbalances can contribute to emotional lability, irritability, and difficulty managing emotions.

Executive Function

Executive functions are an essential set of cognitive skills that act like the brain's "control center," enabling us to navigate daily life effectively. These higher-level thinking abilities allow us to plan, organize, and regulate our behavior, ensuring we can set goals, make decisions, and achieve our objectives (Mutti-Driscoll, 2025). Think of executive functioning as the brain's control room. It guides our thoughts, emotions, and the actions that follow. However, with ADHD, the control room struggles to manage the different parts. This leads to allowing some parts of the brain to run the show (emotions) and others to take a back seat.

If there's one thing these differences show us, it's that the myth that ADHD doesn't exist is completely false. It's not just something people make up to excuse their behavior. It's a genuine condition that shouldn't be dismissed as nothing. There is scientific proof to back up that ADHD is very real. Speaking of myths, let's explore a few other ADHD myths we can debunk.

ADHD Misconceptions and Myths

If you or a loved one are living with ADHD, chances are that you've been confronted with a few ADHD myths and misconceptions. One of the biggest reasons why there are so many misunderstandings about ADHD is due to a lack of education and awareness. Even healthcare professionals are learning more about ADHD every day and may not have all the answers yet. Many people aren't aware of the true nature of ADHD and how it manifests in different individuals, often leading to stereotypes. ADHD is also stigmatized, making ADHDers seem lazy, unmotivated, and undisciplined, leading to a negative belief and attitude about the condition. To help you debunk some of these myths, let's take a look at five of the most common ADHD myths and misconceptions, debunking each with science.

It Only Affects Boys

One of the most common myths regarding ADHD is that it only affects boys. While boys are most frequently diagnosed with ADHD, this significantly underrepresents the number of girls affected (Cornwell, 2023). Unfortunately, girls are often overlooked due to the different ways they present their ADHD symptoms. Girls with ADHD are more likely to present symptoms like inattention, difficulty organizing, and emotional regulation issues, which can be harder to recognize. While we'll chat about this in more detail in the next chapter, it's important to understand that ADHD affects both boys and girls, but the latter are more likely to be overlooked, or their symptoms are mistaken for other conditions (like in Megan's story).

ADHD is Due to Poor Parenting

Parents often experience shame and guilt when their children are diagnosed with ADHD. Because the causes of ADHD are unclear, there is a misconception that ADHD is caused by parenting styles. However, this is absolutely untrue. ADHD is a neurodevelopmental disorder with biological and genetic roots. It's not a result of poor parenting or a lack of discipline, and blaming parents is harmful and ignores the complex interplay of factors contributing to ADHD (Cornwell, 2023). Instead of blaming parents, we should rather focus on supporting and encouraging them. When parents are supported without judgment and shame, they are more likely to speak about ADHD openly and receive the right tools to help their child manage their symptoms more effectively. Blaming the parents also hurts their children. Poor understanding of ADHD can also result in frustration between parent and child, impacting their relationship and dynamic negatively.

ADHD is Attention-Seeking

The number of times I've heard people describe those with ADHD as attention-seeking or dramatic is significant. This accusation can be incredibly hurtful and stop ADHDers from asking for help. These individuals genuinely struggle with focusing, controlling impulses, and regulating emotions (Morin, n.d.). Their behaviors are not deliberate attempts to gain attention, even though attention is often the result. Think of the class clown. Chances are, he's bored and, therefore, entertaining everyone else, drawing attention to himself. However, did he disrupt the class just to get attention? Perhaps not. His disruptive behavior was likely due to his struggles with paying attention, being distracted, and having no interest in the content. Additionally, he might also have interrupted the class because it was physically painful to sit still and listen. Just because he receives attention doesn't mean he is doing it for attention.

ADHD Only Affects Children

Many people often assume that ADHD only affects children, and while it often manifests in childhood, it can also persist into adulthood for many individuals. Adults with ADHD may experience challenges in areas such as work, relationships, and daily life, including difficulties with organization, time management, and emotional regulation (Smith, 2025). However, because of this misconception, many adults never get diagnosed as they assume it can't be ADHD. Instead, they internalize, blaming themselves for their struggles, and get treated for all kinds of other conditions, only leading to more frustration. ADHD can absolutely affect adults; it will just begin to look different. Just because you weren't diagnosed as a child doesn't mean you don't have ADHD as an adult.

You Can Outgrow ADHD

This myth is a continuation of the previous one. While we've confirmed that ADHD doesn't only affect children, it's also necessary to understand that you can't outgrow ADHD. If you were diagnosed as a child, you're not going to suddenly outgrow it or wake up one day with fewer symptoms. ADHD is not something that goes away. However, how it manifests and affects your life might change as your circumstances and responsibilities progress. In other words, some symptoms might lessen with age and with using effective management strategies, but it's a lifelong condition. It may evolve, but it won't evaporate (Cornwell, 2023).

Understanding these realities is important for reducing stigma, improving diagnosis, and providing (or receiving) appropriate support for individuals with ADHD throughout their lives.

Why So Many Tips and Techniques Fail

Chances are, this isn't the first ADHD book you've ever read. You've probably read some articles and other self-help books and probably tried some of the tools and techniques provided in those resources. I've spoken to so many clients who are frustrated and depleted because they've tried tips and techniques marketed to them as ADHD-friendly, only to find they don't work. So, if other techniques have failed, what makes this book different? Unlike most other methods, this approach incorporates two essential components: flexibility and creativity.

Neurotypical tools were designed to work with a neurotypical mind. Yet, we expect it should help those with ADHD, too. In other words, we assume that ADHDers struggle with organization and time management can be solved by a simple technique such as a calendar or a diary. It works for everyone else; why won't it work for ADHDers, right? Wrong. It won't work for ADHDers because the tools weren't designed to work for their specific minds. Basically, we're saying, "Just try harder," which is about as useful as telling someone wearing glasses to "Just see better." Neurotypical tools tend to be linear and rigid, which aren't necessarily things the ADHD brain thrives on. That's why so many tips and techniques you've tried in the past have failed.

The approach of this book will allow you to be flexible and modify every tool provided. Not only will it encourage modification, but it will also provide examples of how to change each tool to better fit the needs of your mind. So, when you're introduced to a tool or technique in this book, see it as an undecorated cake. You get to choose what you want to add or remove to create a "cake" that works for you.

Before we get to customizing techniques, we first need to dive a little deeper into why so many techniques and tips fail. In this chapter, we've learned what ADHD looks like on the inside of the body, and now it's time to look at how it's presented outwardly. Slight spoiler: it looks different in various types of people, and that's why you can't approach ADHD with one-size-fits-all techniques. We'll learn more about that in the next chapter!

Chapter 2:

What Does ADHD Look Like?

ADHD is like going through life, carrying a one-man band contraption with a broken strap. –Julia Smith-Ruetz

I recently had the privilege of working with a set of twins: a boy and a girl. Their parents brought them in to be evaluated after the teacher at school suggested that their son had ADHD. When I met them for the first time, they weren't planning on testing their daughter for ADHD because she was an exemplary child in class. She was quiet, kept to herself, and didn't disrupt the class— unlike her brother. Sure, she struggled with math and sometimes snuck off to the reading corner to have a nap, but she didn't have ADHD. Right? Well, after a brief discussion and explaining to the parents that ADHD looks different in boys and girls, they agreed to have her tested as well.

Both kids were absolutely lovely to work with. They were well-mannered, kind, and unafraid to try new things. But it was very clear to me that both had ADHD. While the boy was a typical hyperactive-impulsive case, the girl was inattentive. They were two sides of the same coin, even though their behavior appeared polar opposite. What stood out to me the most was when I spoke to the girl alone and asked her whether she'd been struggling in certain areas. She nodded her head and elaborated on her struggles. When I asked her why she hadn't told anyone about her, her answer was heartbreaking. She said, "I didn't want to be any trouble or add to my parents' worries."

ADHD can manifest in numerous ways, with each case being unique. While there are some common signs and symptoms of ADHD across different groups of people, it's important to understand that individuals within any group may not experience

ADHD the same. It's simply the most common presentation of ADHD in the discussed group. In this chapter, we'll look at how ADHD can present differently in these specific groups, including males, females, children, and adults. Before then, it's worth taking a look at how ADHD is perceived by different generations.

ADHD Through the Generations

The way ADHD is perceived by the public has significantly changed in the last couple of decades. When I was still a student in school, most people believed that ADHD wasn't real and that children were just misbehaving and required more discipline. It was difficult to get diagnosed, and parents were often offended when teachers suggested such a diagnosis. As the years have gone by and research has improved, ADHD is a more accepted diagnosis, especially with all the advocacy on social media platforms. But has it changed how people view ADHD? For some, definitely. But the older generations still struggle to wrap their heads around it.

The Older Generations

A lot of the older generations, like Baby Boomers and Gen X, still view ADHD through a lens shaped by limited understanding and the societal norms of their time. Many didn't receive sympathy and support for their struggles with ADHD, and believe they turned out "fine," so they feel that modern children shouldn't be "babied" either. Unfortunately, their views of ADHD are created by a lack of awareness. Since ADHD wasn't widely recognized or understood as a neurodevelopmental disorder in the past, they continue to see it as something that should be dismissed or disciplined. Due to this lack of understanding, ADHD is still sometimes stigmatized as a character flaw or a sign of weakness in their eyes.

The older generations also have a different treatment approach than some of the younger generations. Treatment is often centered on behavior modification techniques rather than addressing the underlying neurological differences. This could involve strict discipline, punishment, and social isolation. Unfortunately, these methods can often do more harm than good. While it can be frustrating to change the stoic mind of the older generation, it's important to also understand that many of them grew up in environments with different expectations and less emphasis on individual needs.

A client of mine, Sandra, faced a lot of backlash from her parents when her son was diagnosed with ADHD. They often said hurtful things to her and to her son, disregarding his needs. Eventually, she had to sit them down and set boundaries. She explained to them that if they didn't get on board and take the time to learn what ADHD really is and how they can support her son, they were no longer welcome in their lives. Although she understood they didn't grow up with ADHD as an acceptable diagnosis or weren't even aware of its existence, she made it clear that they either had to change or face the consequences. While it was an incredibly hard conversation, later that night, they phoned her with questions about ADHD and expressed their interest in attending her son's next clinic appointment to gain more understanding. As they learned more about ADHD, their behavior toward her and her son changed completely.

It's important to have patience and sympathy for those who don't understand ADHD, but that doesn't mean you're not allowed to create a boundary to protect yourself or your loved ones.

The Younger Generations

Unlike the older generations, the younger ones have mostly accepted ADHD as a diagnosis and are more aware of ADHD due to increased research, education, and media coverage. There are thousands of resources dedicated to educating people on ADHD and what it might look like. However, the recent surge in advocacy is a double-edged sword. While it's wonderful that so many people are aware of ADHD, it has become a bit of a trend, often leading to misdiagnosis or overdiagnosis. The younger generation sometimes uses ADHD to describe their quirks rather than viewing it as a serious diagnosis. As an example, when they lose their keys, they might say, "I'm being so ADHD today." Unfortunately, this has led to many misunderstanding the serious impact that ADHD has on daily life and that it goes beyond just losing keys or being late to a party.

I recently saw a video on TikTok with the caption, "If you have any of these symptoms, you have ADHD." The video then proceeded to explain some ADHD symptoms but without the depth necessary to provide accurate information. In other words, it ended up being a list of things ALL human beings experience, such as losing your wallet, getting annoyed with your spouse, or forgetting to do the laundry. While all of these can be attributed to ADHD, they can also be normal human experiences. Additionally, some of my clients have shared that they have been advised by others to just list all the ADHD symptoms when consulting a healthcare professional in order to get diagnosed with ADHD and receive medication. This can be very dangerous, especially if you are listing symptoms you don't actually experience.

It's imperative that we find a balance between the older and younger generations. Ideally, we should all be educated on ADHD and have an understanding of what it is without jumping to self-diagnosis or using it as an excuse. With that in mind, approach the rest of this chapter without trying to self-diagnose or diagnose someone you know. Instead, view it as an opportunity to become more aware of what ADHD might typically look like in different individuals. Even if you have one or two of these symptoms, it doesn't mean that you have ADHD. There are many other conditions with similar symptoms, which we'll talk about in a later chapter. For now, let's focus on how ADHD might present differently in children.

ADHD in Children

Children often display ADHD symptoms differently than adults. This is not because ADHD changes or evolves but because children haven't necessarily learned to mask their behavior to appear "normal," and they have yet to learn effective coping strategies. In other words, they express themselves more outwardly, while adults learn to manage and control those impulse reactions. According to research from 2022, it's estimated that 11.4% of all U.S. children aged 3 to 17 have ADHD (CDC, 2024). That's a significant number, which is why it's especially important to spot ADHD in our children and provide them with the necessary resources and support. However, identifying ADHD in children isn't always easy, especially since it can present very differently in boys and girls.

Boys vs. Girls

ADHD is not necessarily sex-specific. Not all boys have hyperactive-impulsive ADHD, and not all girls have inattentive ADHD. However, the majority of boys present with the hyperactive-impulsive (or combined) type, while it's more common for girls to present as inattentive. For this reason, girls often go undiagnosed for long periods of time. According to studies, boys are three times more likely to be diagnosed with ADHD than girls (Kinman, 2016). However, this doesn't mean that girls are less susceptible to ADHD than boys. Many girls tend to go undiagnosed due to their subtle symptoms.

Boys with ADHD most commonly show externalized symptoms, such as running around and acting impulsively. On the other hand, girls show more internalized symptoms, such as low self-esteem and inattentiveness to details. We know that ADHD can play a big role in emotions, and children don't necessarily have the right tools to manage this rollercoaster ride yet. So, how do they deal with their frustration? Boys with ADHD tend to behave physically aggressively to get rid of their anger, while girls rely on verbal expressions (Kinman, 2016). Unfortunately, this leads to girls being labeled as "snarky" or "catty" instead of seeing it as a sign of ADHD.

Because ADHD in girls often goes unnoticed, they may not receive the treatment and support they need. This further pressures them to "be better," adding tremendous weight to be perfect all the time. While boys are more likely to receive proper treatment and learn coping strategies, girls are subconsciously taught to hide it from the world without showing any struggles, leading to a negative impact on their self-esteem and mental health. Girls with ADHD are also more likely to turn their pain and anger inward, which can result in depression, anxiety, and eating disorders.

To clearly see the difference in how boys and girls typically differ in their ADHD presentation, let's take a look at these two tables. Remember, this is a generalization, and every child should still be treated individually. Some girls might present more like the symptoms listed as common for boys, and vice versa.

Common ADHD Symptoms in Girls
withdrawing from others and keeping to oneself
low self-esteem and confidence
anxiety and stress over seemingly small things
overwhelm easily
struggles with academic achievement
tendency to daydream
struggles with focusing on important matters
zoning out while others are talking (It's more entertaining to create their own scenarios)
verbal aggression, such as taunting and name-calling

Common ADHD Symptoms in Boys
acting impulsively
acting out in class and at home
unable to sit still and tend to give up easily
lack of focus in serious settings

interpersonal conflicts with others
physical aggression as a way to solve problems
talking excessively
interrupting other people's conversations and activities
unable to wait their turn; frequently taking over an activity from someone else

ADHD in Adults

As ADHD children mature, whether diagnosed or not, their symptoms often begin to change. For example, a child who used to run around the classroom and disrupt everyone might now present as being restless, having difficulty relaxing, and talking excessively. Impulsivity can grow into struggles with decision-making, risk-taking, and strong emotional outbursts. Inattention can manifest as difficulty focusing and completing work, forgetfulness, and disorganization. In other words, your ADHD doesn't go away once you hit 18 or 21, but it can present differently.

One reason why ADHD symptoms appear to change is that adults learn to mask their feelings and adopt behaviors they believe are acceptable to others. It's like an elaborate game of play-pretend where you're trying to fit in with those around you. This can lead to severe burnout as tremendous amounts of energy are required to keep this up. It can also lead to imposter syndrome and mental health issues since you'll always feel like being yourself isn't good enough.

A client of mine, Janet, once shared with me how exhausting it was for her to be around her in-laws. "I always have to pretend like I'm better than I am," she explained. "I grew up in a home where my mom allowed me to walk barefoot and laugh loudly. Now I feel like I have to keep myself settled," she shared. In other words, Janet felt like she was riding a horse that she had to keep at a walking pace when she knew all the horse wanted was to run.

Masking can be helpful in certain situations, especially in professional settings. But it's not a viable long-term solution. Instead of pretending, we should focus on finding tools and techniques that allow us to effectively manage our struggles rather than pretending they don't exist. Managing techniques is another reason why ADHD symptoms might appear differently in adults than in children. Chances are, somewhere in your life, you learned that visibly zoning out while someone is talking to you doesn't sit well with the other person. So, you've learned to look away or focus on something else while the person is talking, which helps you better process and hear what they're saying.

Symptoms also evolve with age as we mature. Brad might no longer push his friend away to get a turn on the golf course, like he did back in kindergarten by the swings. However, he might still make a snarky remark about how long his friend is taking to take the shot. Either way, he's still struggling with waiting his turn; it's just presented differently. If an outsider saw Brad's behavior, they wouldn't assume he had ADHD—they might simply assume he's being rude or arrogant.

Men and Women

Men and Women can often have different presentations of ADHD symptoms, and the same differences that begin in childhood will continue as ADHDers get older. Men tend to be more impulsive and might even partake in reckless behaviors

(ADDA Editorial Team, 2023). This includes driving fast, substance abuse, taking shortcuts, and hobbies that can be dangerous. They are also more likely to make decisions on a whim. This always reminds me of a scene in the TV series *Modern Family*, where Phil comes home with an alpaca. Why? Because he saw it, and it was the very last one for sale. Impulsivity in men doesn't necessarily always result in coming home from the store with cute animals. It can also mean being reckless with finances, such as gambling or making expensive purchases that weren't needed (like a speedboat).

ADHD in women is a continuation of how it is presented in childhood. Women are more likely to showcase symptoms such as forgetfulness, disorganization, and difficulty focusing. They are also most likely struggling with other mental issues due to a lack of proper treatment and the habit of internalizing every perceived failure. This includes mental struggles such as depression and anxiety. Women with ADHD might also become more irritable with others and overly self-critical. In general, they are very hard on themselves since they learned from a young age that struggling with normal day activities is their own fault. Women with ADHD can also face more overwhelming struggles than men, such as looking after the family, children, chores, work, and other demands.

ADHD in both adult men and women often leads to jumping from hobby to hobby. Chances are, if you have ADHD, there's a good chance you have a cupboard filled with equipment and supplies for hobbies you've completely forgotten about or have given up before trying. A lot of behavior in adults with ADHD is motivated by seeking a dopamine rush since their bodies have lower dopamine levels, making it harder for them to stay engaged.

Understanding these differences is crucial when it comes to diagnosis and management strategies. Some techniques might be geared toward helping the typical man with ADHD, while others might be geared more suited to women. However, don't assume that all men and women's symptoms will always fit into these exact categories. As mentioned before, these are generalizations, but every case should be treated uniquely.

Checklist With ADHD Symptoms

As I mentioned earlier, the goal of this book isn't to self-diagnose but to educate, equip, and empower. However, it can be very helpful to evaluate your own behavior and see how it aligns with ADHD symptoms to get a better idea of whether further testing is required. The following questions have been designed to help you your thoughts and behaviors to identify whether some of the struggles you've been experiencing might actually be symptoms of ADHD.

I once helped a client, Jessica, work through this list, and by the end, she was in tears. "I always thought I was just bad at these things. I never realized they were actually part of my ADHD," she said. Even if these questions simply make you feel seen, they've done their job. Take a look at these questions and take your time to answer each one truthfully. You don't have to pretend to be perfect here—just be your glorious self.

The first set of questions is aimed at inattentive ADHD symptoms.

- Do you find it challenging to remain attentive during tasks that require sustained mental effort, such as reading, attending work meetings, or watching a movie?

- Do you easily get distracted by irrelevant stimuli, such as noise, movement, or your own thoughts?

- Do you often feel like your mind is racing or that you have too many random thoughts going on at once?

- Are you frequently forgetful of appointments, deadlines, or important events?

- Do you often lose or misplace important items (e.g., keys, wallet, phone, documents)?

- Do you struggle with time management and often find yourself late or running behind schedule?

- Do you sometimes feel like you have a lot of time but end up running out of time due to a lack of awareness?

- Is your workspace, home, or digital environment cluttered and disorganized?

- Do you often try to work on improving your organizational skills but never complete any tasks?

- Do you have trouble completing tasks that require sustained effort, such as household chores, work projects, or long-term goals?

- Do you often feel overwhelmed by the prospect of starting a new task or project?

- Do you tend to procrastinate or avoid tasks that require sustained attention?

- Do you often feel inadequate, incompetent, or like you don't measure up?

- Do you experience frequent feelings of frustration, anxiety, or low self-worth?

The following questions are aimed at hyperactive and impulsive symptoms.

- Do you often feel restless or fidgety, even when you're trying to relax?

- Do you find it difficult to sit still for extended periods, such as during meetings or while traveling?

- Do you often feel like you have excess energy that you can't seem to channel?

- Do you often act on impulse without thinking things through?

- Do you often interrupt others or find it difficult to wait your turn?

- Do you engage in risky behaviors, such as reckless driving, impulsive spending, or substance abuse?

- Do you have trouble maintaining close friendships or romantic relationships?

- Do you often experience conflict in your relationships due to impulsivity, irritability, or difficulty communicating?

- Do you have difficulty managing your emotions, such as anger, frustration, or sadness?

- Do you experience frequent mood swings or emotional outbursts?

As this chapter comes to a close, take some time to process your answers to these questions. If you said yes to most of them, your behavior and thoughts are similar to someone with ADHD, and it's worth investigating it further, particularly if it impacts your day-to-day functioning. In the next chapter, we'll continue this pursuit of unpacking ADHD as we explore the various ways in which it can impact your life.

Chapter 3:

The Impact of ADHD on Your Life

ADHD is having the day off and thinking of 1,000 ways to enjoy it, deciding on none of those, and frozen by your own inability to choose an activity. -Rene Brooks

"I can't have ADHD because I don't struggle to sit still, and I do well in school." As someone who works with ADHD clients on a daily basis, this is something I hear quite often. Many people know about ADHD and understand that it's real, but there's still a big gap in educating the public on how it can impact a person's life. ADHD doesn't only affect one area. It's not like you struggle with ADHD at work and are unaffected at home. ADHD isn't only contained to one area of your life; rather, it can impact every area, sometimes in ways you don't even realize. Because it's all you know, you assume that's how it's supposed to be. Doesn't everyone struggle to keep in touch with close friends and not completely ghost them for months at a time? Well, not really.

It's vital to be aware of all the areas of your life that are impacted by ADHD so you can implement the right strategies and tools to help them. For example, if you're not aware that ADHD can impact your social life, you'll never think to create a system that will allow you to manage your symptoms in order to improve your social life. In this chapter, we'll look at four main areas affected by ADHD: academic life and work-life, social and interpersonal relationships, mental and emotional well-being, and daily life and practical challenges.

Academic Life and Work-Life

ADHD presents unique challenges in academic and professional settings, but it can also offer some distinct strengths. That said, I'm not trying to downplay the significant impact ADHD can have on someone's life. I'm also not going to call ADHD a "superpower" since I believe that highly diminishes the impact ADHD can have on you. However, if there's an upside, even a small one, it's important for your well-being that you are aware of it and choose to focus on it as well. We shouldn't only focus on the negative or positives but rather on how to approach it with objectivity and clarity.

Challenges

I recently spoke to a client of mine who has been struggling with his academic studies at university. After explaining to him how ADHD can impact every area of his life, including academics, he paused and said, "Wait, this isn't something everyone struggles with?" ADHDers often get so used to the daily struggles that they don't recognize when those struggles are actually ADHD-related. In this section, we will explore how ADHD can manifest in academic and work life, examining the difficulties you may encounter in areas like focus, organization, and time management.

Organization, Time Management, and Prioritization

For ADHDers, organization, time management, and prioritization can pose significant challenges in both academic and professional settings. Difficulty with organization can manifest in cluttered workspaces, misplaced items, and a general sense of disarray. This disorganization can extend to academic tasks, leading to missed assignments, difficulty locating necessary materials, and a lack of structure in study habits (Green, 2023). Time management often proves problematic due to impulsivity and distractibility. Procrastination becomes a common coping mechanism, as focusing on a task for an extended period can feel overwhelming. This can result in missed deadlines, incomplete projects, and a general feeling of being constantly behind (Niermann & Scheres, 2014).

Another major hurdle for those with ADHD in their academic and work lives is prioritizing tasks effectively. ADHDers may struggle to identify the most important tasks, leading to them getting sidetracked by less urgent but more stimulating activities. This can lead to a feeling of being overwhelmed and a sense of never accomplishing anything meaningful. These challenges can significantly impact academic and professional success, leading to frustration, low self-esteem, and difficulties in maintaining a healthy work-life balance. Some people with ADHD might find they are able to focus at work due to the nature of their work, being stimulated, or experiencing frequent changes. However, they might then struggle with organization and prioritization in their family life after work as they have exhausted their mental capacity at work.

Sustained Attention

Sustained attention is the ability to focus on a task for an extended period of time. If you're not familiar with what that feels like, you're not alone. Sustained focus is a significant challenge for individuals with ADHD due to neurological differences (Cleveland Clinic, 2023a). The ADHD brain affects the ability to filter out distractions, which means sustained focus doesn't come easily or often. As a result, ADHDers may experience difficulty concentrating on lectures, reading assignments, or completing tasks that require prolonged focus.

This can lead to frustration, decreased productivity, and difficulties in academic and professional settings.

A student with ADHD might find it challenging to focus on a lengthy textbook chapter. Their mind may wander to other thoughts or be easily distracted by noises in the environment. This can make it difficult to absorb information and retain it for later recall. Similarly, in a workplace setting, an employee with ADHD might struggle to complete a detailed report, finding their attention drawn to emails, social media notifications, or conversations around them. There can be errors, missed deadlines, and a decrease in job satisfaction as a result.

Written Assignments, Note-Taking, and Completing Projects

For ADHDers, written assignments can be a major obstacle in their work and academic life. The act of putting thoughts onto paper can be daunting, with their mind easily wandering off to other, seemingly more interesting topics. This can lead to procrastination and difficulty in starting and finishing assignments. Additionally, the organizational aspect of writing, such as structuring ideas and creating outlines, can be overwhelming, which can result in messy, disorganized work that lacks clarity and coherence (Molitor et al., 2016). Those diagnosed with ADHD are often accused of not caring about their work due to this exact reason, even though it's not something they do on purpose.

Another challenge lies in note-taking, especially in a traditional classroom setting. The constant stream of information can be very overwhelming, making it hard to focus on the key points (James, 2024). Additionally, distractions, both internal and external, can easily derail the note-taking process. This can lead to incomplete or inaccurate notes, which can hinder learning and comprehension. Both note-taking and writing assignments are usually necessary to complete projects, which is why project completion is another major obstacle for ADHDers. The long-term nature of projects can be overwhelming, making it difficult to break them down into manageable steps.

Academic Underachievement and Career Instability

For those with ADHD, the challenges of academic underachievement and career instability can significantly impact their lives. Academically, ADHD symptoms like difficulty focusing, organizing tasks, and managing time can lead to lower grades, missed deadlines, and difficulty completing assignments. This can create a cycle of frustration and discouragement, further hindering academic progress (Adamou et al., 2013).

In the workplace, ADHD can manifest as challenges with maintaining focus during meetings, prioritizing tasks, and meeting deadlines. This can lead to difficulties in building and maintaining professional relationships, impacting career advancement. Because of this, ADHDers are more likely to experience increased job dissatisfaction and higher rates of job turnover (Adamou et al., 2013). An ADHDer might excel in their field but struggle to manage their time effectively. This could lead to missed deadlines, incomplete projects, and, ultimately, job instability.

While these challenges might feel overwhelming, with the right tools and techniques, every person managing their ADHD can learn to navigate their symptoms and thrive in the workplace and in academic pursuits—especially once they learn how to harness their strengths.

Strengths

As we explore the cognitive strengths often associated with ADHD, such as creativity, hyperfocus, and the ability to think outside the box, it's important to be mindful of the challenges you face. Why? When you have a specific challenge in mind, but you're aware of your strengths, you can start building mental tools to address it effectively. By understanding both the difficulties and strengths of ADHD, you can develop effective coping strategies and leverage your unique talents to succeed in your academic and professional endeavors.

Creativity and Innovation

Many individuals with ADHD possess a unique blend of traits that can fuel creativity and innovation. You might not consider yourself creative in the sense of arts and crafts, but that doesn't mean you can't be creative in other ways (such as problem-solving). The ADHD mind tends to wander and make unexpected connections, leading to novel ideas and solutions (Bozhilova et al., 2018). This can be particularly beneficial in fields that value out-of-the-box thinking, such as entrepreneurship and scientific research. For example, an individual with ADHD might brainstorm a new marketing campaign by associating seemingly unrelated concepts, resulting in a highly original and effective strategy.

The impulsivity associated with ADHD can sometimes be channeled into a fearless pursuit of new ideas. In other words, ADHDers can turn a weakness into a strength, leading to a willingness to take risks and experiment, which is essential for groundbreaking innovation (Kelly, n.d.). In a workplace setting, an individual with ADHD might propose a radical new approach to a problem, even if it challenges the status quo. This willingness to challenge norms can drive progress and lead to significant breakthroughs.

Hyperfocus

Hyperfocus is a state of intense concentration that most ADHDers are familiar with. It involves becoming deeply engrossed in a specific task or activity, often for extended periods (Think ADHD, 2024). While it can sometimes be disruptive, hyperfocus can also be a significant strength, particularly in academic and work settings. When channeled effectively, hyperfocus can lead to remarkable productivity and creativity. Those individuals with ADHD who hyperfocus can often achieve a high level of output and produce exceptional results in their chosen fields. This intense focus allows them to investigate complex problems, explore intricate details, and generate innovative solutions.

For example, a student diagnosed with ADHD might hyperfocus on a particularly engaging research project. They might spend hours pouring over academic articles, conducting experiments, and analyzing data with unwavering dedication. This intense focus can lead to groundbreaking discoveries and an in-depth understanding of the subject matter. Similarly, hyperfocus can be a valuable asset at work (Think ADHD, 2024). When engaged in a task that captures their interest, ADHDers can demonstrate exceptional problem-solving skills, meticulous attention to detail, and unwavering determination. This focused energy can drive them to excel in their roles and contribute significantly to their teams.

Enthusiasm and Drive to Succeed

Individuals with ADHD often possess a unique blend of enthusiasm and drive that can be a significant asset in both academic and professional settings. When immersed in a subject or task that captures their interest, they can exhibit remarkable focus, energy, and determination. This passion can fuel late nights of study, inspire innovative solutions, and drive them to excel in their chosen fields (*The 5 Things Proven to*, 2024).

This inherent drive can be particularly beneficial in fast-paced or dynamic environments where adaptability and a proactive approach are valued. For example, an entrepreneur with ADHD might leverage their intense focus and creative problem-solving abilities to identify a niche market and develop a successful business model. Their enthusiasm can be contagious, motivating colleagues and fostering a collaborative spirit within a team.

Social and Interpersonal Relationships

Another area of life adversely affected by ADHD is social and interpersonal relationships. ADHD can present both unique and unexpected challenges in this area of life, and this section will explore how that might look. There are both challenges and strengths associated with ADHD, but one doesn't nullify the other. You can embrace the strengths without ignoring the severity of the challenges. It's valuable to consider both as they will help you find solutions that actually work for your ADHD mind. Let's start by exploring the challenges of social and interpersonal relationships and ADHD.

Challenges

Many ADHDers don't realize that their social and interpersonal relationships are affected by their ADHD. According to research, ADHD can severely impact the quality and quantity of your relationships (*Relationships & Social Skills*, 2018). While it's important to be aware of these challenges, people with ADHD should be careful not to fall into the trap of self-fulfilled prophecy. This can occur when you are so focused on your challenges that you believe it's impossible to have a healthy relationship, so you behave in a way that pushes others away. At that point, it is no longer your ADHD that serves as the challenge but rather your belief that there is nothing you can do about it. Let's explore the main challenges that ADHDers might experience in this area.

Maintaining Friendships and Romantic Relationships

Many individuals with ADHD face unique challenges in maintaining friendships and romantic relationships. Their forgetfulness and disorganization can lead to missed appointments, forgotten promises, and a lack of follow-through on plans, which can strain relationships over time. Additionally, their impulsivity may lead to outbursts or risky behaviors that can damage trust and intimacy (Normand et al., 2007).

Furthermore, the hyperfocus associated with ADHD can sometimes make it difficult to maintain a healthy balance between personal relationships and other interests. When deeply engrossed in a hobby or project, someone with ADHD might neglect social commitments, leading to feelings of resentment or abandonment from their partners. This can create a cycle of guilt and frustration for both parties involved. Some ADHDers also find it draining to initiate contact with peers as they don't like small talk.

Impulsivity Leading to Conflicts

Impulsivity can be a significant challenge for those with ADHD, particularly in social and interpersonal relationships. It can lead to unintended consequences and strain relationships with loved ones (Jordan, 2024). For example, a person with ADHD might impulsively blurt out something hurtful or insensitive without considering the impact on the other person. This can lead to hurt feelings, arguments, and strained relationships. Impulsivity can also manifest in other ways, such as interrupting others, making snap judgments, or acting without thinking. This can make it difficult for individuals with ADHD to maintain healthy relationships and can lead to feelings of isolation and loneliness.

Emotional Regulation

Since ADHDers find it hard to manage and respond to their emotions, it can often lead to unexpected behavior and outbursts. This can be very frustrating for the other parties involved, especially when they expect the ADHDers to share with them as freely. Poor emotional regulation can also lead to difficulty reading social cues and struggles with empathy. Friendships, family relationships, and romantic relationships can be strained by these challenges. For example, a person with ADHD might struggle to control their frustration when faced with a minor inconvenience, leading to an outburst that could damage a relationship. They might also have difficulty understanding or responding appropriately to the emotions of others, leading to misunderstandings and hurt feelings. This can make it difficult to build and maintain deep, meaningful connections with others.

Listening and Maintaining Eye Contact

Listening and maintaining eye contact can be significant challenges in social and interpersonal relationships for someone diagnosed with ADHD. This is largely due to the core symptoms of ADHD, which include inattention, impulsivity, and hyperactivity. When engaged in a conversation, those individuals with ADHD may find it difficult to filter out extraneous stimuli, leading to distractions and difficulty focusing on the speaker (Novotni, 2021). This can manifest as zoning out during conversations, missing key points, or frequently interrupting.

Specifically, maintaining eye contact can be a struggle because it can feel overwhelming to the ADHDers. While it's usually a sign of engagement and respect, intense and direct eye contact can feel intrusive to those with ADHD (Novotni, 2024). This can inadvertently convey disinterest or disengagement to the other person, hindering the development of meaningful connections. For example, imagine a person with ADHD in a job interview. They may find it challenging to maintain eye contact with the interviewer while simultaneously processing their questions and formulating thoughtful responses. This could lead to them appearing unfocused or even evasive, potentially negatively impacting their chances of securing the position.

Strengths

With all the difficulties, socializing might feel overwhelming for someone with ADHD. What's the point in trying if you'll never get it right? Well, that's why it's vital to also focus on the strengths. They won't remove the challenges, but they will allow you to shift your focus to all the wonderful things you add to social situations and relationships. While there are challenges, you can overcome them and foster long-lasting, healthy relationships, especially with the help of these strengths.

Empathy

Individuals with ADHD often possess a heightened capacity for empathy, which can be a significant strength in their social and interpersonal relationships. This enhanced empathy may stem from their own experiences navigating the challenges of ADHD, fostering a deeper understanding of others' struggles and sensitivities (ADDitude Editors, 2024). For example, those who have ADHD might be particularly attuned to the emotional needs of a friend experiencing anxiety, offering support and understanding in a way that someone without ADHD might not.

This heightened empathy can create strong bonds and foster deep, meaningful connections with others.

Energy and Enthusiasm in Social Situations

Many ADHDers possess a unique blend of energy and enthusiasm that can be a significant asset in social situations. When engaged in a conversation or activity that captures their interest, they can be incredibly animated, bringing a vibrant energy to the interaction. This enthusiasm can be contagious, drawing others in and creating a dynamic and engaging atmosphere (Holmes, 2024). Such inherent energy can be particularly beneficial in group settings, where it can spark creativity and encourage active participation. For example, an individual with ADHD might be the life of a party, effortlessly engaging with others and fostering a sense of camaraderie. Their passion for a particular topic can also inspire others to learn and explore new ideas, leading to stimulating and enriching conversations.

Humor

The ADHD mind tends to make unexpected connections, which can lead to witty observations and offbeat jokes that can surprise and delight those around them. This ability to find humor in everyday situations can be a powerful tool for building rapport and creating a lighthearted atmosphere (Smith, 2025). For example, a person with ADHD might use their hyperfocus to notice a small detail in a conversation and then weave it into a humorous anecdote that leaves their listener chuckling. This ability to think outside the box can also make them skilled at improvisation, allowing them to adapt quickly to changing social situations and use humor to navigate awkward moments with grace.

Mental and Emotional Well-Being

In recent years, there's been a lot of advocacy and information regarding emotional and mental well-being. This has brought a lot of attention to how ADHD and other disorders can affect one's overall mental health and well-being. It's absolutely essential for everyone to take care of their mental health, especially ADHDers. Due to the emotional rollercoaster that ADHD often causes, it's normal for an individual's mental health to suffer. When you constantly experience ups and downs of emotions, it can be exhausting and quite debilitating. Being aware of the challenges and the strengths that ADHD has on mental and emotional well-being is a great first step in taking care of your mental health. By understanding your own mental and emotional well-being and how ADHD can affect it, you will be better equipped to create the right systems to help with emotional management.

Challenges

Life can be hard, and it can lead to many mental and emotional challenges, regardless of whether you have ADHD or not. With all the challenges humans face on a daily basis and with increased pressure to be perfect, it's no wonder that ADHD can impact your emotional well-being so deeply. Let's explore three ways in which ADHD can contribute to this already challenging area of life.

Anxiety and Depression

Anxiety and depression commonly occur in people with ADHD. ADHD symptoms, such as difficulty concentrating and impulsivity, can lead to feelings of inadequacy and frustration.

These feelings can then contribute to the development of anxiety and depression (Katzman et al., 2017). For example, a person with ADHD may worry excessively about making mistakes at work, feeling as though their efforts are never good enough, leading to increased anxiety and a decrease in self-esteem. The result can then be a downward spiral, as the person's anxiety and depression make it even more difficult to manage their ADHD symptoms.

Substance Abuse

Substance abuse is another common mental health challenge for people with ADHD, as difficulties with control impulses can lead to problems with substance abuse. People with ADHD may also use substances to self-medicate their symptoms (Watson, 2024). For example, someone with ADHD may use alcohol or cannabis to help them relax and fall asleep. However, alcohol can actually worsen ADHD symptoms and make it more difficult to manage the condition.

Sleep Disturbances

Sleep disturbances are also common among people with ADHD, making it difficult to fall asleep and stay asleep (Hvolby, 2014). This can be due to racing thoughts, difficulty winding down, or restlessness. Sleep problems can then exacerbate ADHD symptoms, making it even more difficult to concentrate and control impulses. For example, a person with ADHD may have trouble falling asleep at night because they are constantly thinking about the things they need to do the next day or other random thoughts. This can lead to a vicious cycle of sleep deprivation and worsening ADHD symptoms.

Strengths

The perception of mental well-being varies from person to person. For some, managing mental health might mean taking a break from social media or searching for a new job. However, there are some ADHD traits that can help in this area of life. While these traits aren't exclusive to ADHDers, they are more likely to exhibit these qualities. Here are three examples of how having ADHD can help in taking care of mental health.

Resilience

Individuals with ADHD can exhibit remarkable resilience in the face of challenges (Dangmann et al., 2024). Their experiences often necessitate a high degree of adaptability and problem-solving, fostering a strong sense of resourcefulness. For example, those diagnosed with ADHD might have to develop creative strategies for managing time and staying organized, leading to a greater ability to navigate unexpected obstacles and bounce back from setbacks.

Imagination

Imagination is another notable strength often found in someone with ADHD. Their minds often operate in a state of heightened awareness, leading to vivid inner worlds and a unique perspective on the world around them. This can manifest in a strong sense of creativity, whether it be in artistic pursuits, problem-solving, or simply finding innovative ways to approach everyday tasks (*How Does ADHD Impact Problem*, 2024). For example, an individual with ADHD might use their vivid imagination to develop a new and exciting approach to a challenging project, leading to a novel and unexpected outcome.

Embracing Spontaneity

Embracing spontaneity can be a true gift for those with ADHD. Their natural inclination toward flexibility and adaptability can make them more open to new experiences and opportunities. This can lead to a richer, more fulfilling life filled with unexpected adventures and joyful discoveries. For example, an individual with ADHD might be more likely to seize a last-minute opportunity for travel or a spontaneous social gathering, leading to a memorable and enriching experience.

Daily Life and Practical Challenges

Besides the challenges we've already discussed, ADHD also poses a number of practical challenges in daily life. Things that neurotypicals find easy might be very challenging for ADHDers. This can lead to all sorts of other issues, including exhaustion and burnout. It's important to be aware of these challenges so you'll know which areas to focus on when you're choosing tools to implement into your life. For example, if you know that you struggle with keeping a routine, you'll know to search for a tool that will specifically help you create a routine that works for your ADHD mind. It's equally important to know what your strengths are so you can use them in crafting the tools.

Challenges

There are all kinds of challenges that come with ADHD, but let's focus on two specific challenges that most ADHDers find frustrating.

Routines

Someone with ADHD can find it really challenging to establish and maintain consistent routines. That's because their minds crave novelty and spontaneity, making the repetition of daily tasks feel monotonous and uninspiring. This can lead to difficulty with tasks like waking up on time, completing chores, or sticking to a regular sleep schedule. For example, a person with ADHD might set an alarm for work but then find themselves easily distracted by social media, leading to a late start to the day and a feeling of being behind from the outset.

Losing Personal Belongings

The inattention and distractibility that are hallmark symptoms of ADHD can make it easy for an individual to misplace their personal belongings. A person might set their keys down in one location, only to find themselves frantically searching for them later on. This tendency can extend to larger items as well, such as wallets, phones, or even important documents. For example, a student with ADHD might place their backpack down while studying, only to realize later that they have no idea where they put it, leading to a stressful search before an important class.

Strengths

There's one key strength that ADHD brings to the table that shouldn't be overlooked. It's often seen as a weakness or something the ADHD mind craves, but it can also be a strength.

Flexibility

Individuals with ADHD often possess remarkable flexibility and adaptability. Their minds are wired to adjust quickly to unexpected changes and find alternative solutions when faced with obstacles. This agility can be a significant asset in dynamic environments, allowing them to thrive in situations where rigid routines would be detrimental. For example, a project manager who has been diagnosed with ADHD might excel at navigating unforeseen challenges, seamlessly reprioritizing tasks, and adjusting schedules to ensure project success.

Understanding the impact of ADHD on everyday life is fundamental for individuals with ADHD and those who interact with them. By acknowledging both the challenges and strengths associated with ADHD, individuals can develop effective coping strategies, cultivate their unique talents, and build fulfilling lives. Recognizing ADHD's effects can lead to increased self-awareness, improved self-compassion, and a greater understanding of personal strengths and weaknesses. This knowledge can empower individuals to advocate for themselves, seek appropriate support, and build a life that aligns with their unique neurodiversity.

In the next chapter, we'll continue this journey of unpacking ADHD by examining other mental health conditions that often overlap with it. If you need a break from this information-heavy chapter, feel free to take one. But remember to set a reminder for when you want to return so you don't forget.

Chapter 4:

ADHD and Other Mental Health Conditions

My ADHD makes me like a phone on shuffle. You never know what's coming next. - Anonymous

One of the biggest misconceptions about ADHD is that it's an isolated condition. The truth is that ADHD is often associated with other comorbidities. What does that mean? Comorbidity is a medical term that means the simultaneous presence of two or more medical conditions in one patient (Cleveland Clinic, 2024a). It's a complex phenomenon that is influenced by a variety of factors, including genetics, lifestyle, and environmental exposures. It also makes diagnosing and treating patients much harder since symptoms can often overlap.

On this ADHD journey, it's important to be aware of overlapping conditions because not all symptoms in your life that "sound" like ADHD are a definite sign that you have ADHD. Due to the complex nature of comorbid conditions, many symptoms that appear to be one thing might actually be a sign of something else. In this chapter, we'll explore how ADHD presents alongside various other conditions, including depression, personality disorders, autism, and many more. Similar to the previous chapter, the goal is not to diagnose you with one or the other. Rather, it's to get to know yourself and be aware that there might be some things to investigate further. It will also allow you to know where to start on your ADHD management journey. On that note, let's jump right in, starting with ADHD and oppositional defiant disorder.

ADHD and Oppositional Defiant Disorder

Oppositional defiant disorder (ODD) is defined by aggressive behavior and a persistent pattern of hostile and vindictive behavior toward authority figures. Children with ODD will often annoy adults and peers in authoritative positions on purpose and will become irritable and argumentative when given orders from an authoritative figure (ADDtitude Editors, 2019). ODD can begin in childhood or adolescence, and it can progress into worse disorders when left untreated. Similarly to ADHD, the symptoms of ODD may look different in boys and girls. Boys tend to present more physically aggressive with explosive episodes of anger, while girls might lie and refuse to cooperate. Unlike ADHD, you can grow out of ODD, and it's not a lifelong condition.

According to studies, 40% of children with ADHD also experience ODD (ADDtitude Editors, 2021). However, not all children with ODD have ADHD, and not everyone with ADHD has ODD. The aggressive behavior of ODD, combined with the impulsivity of ADHD, can be a volatile combination, leading to intense arguments and even physical violence. Children with ADHD might also have more energy than other children, which, combined with the physical nature of ODD, can lead to roughhousing and harm to their peers (Higuera, 2019). Since both conditions involve issues with controlling impulses and emotions, the lines can become blurred when trying to determine which disorder is causing what behavior.

Symptoms of ODD include (ADDtitude Editors, 2019):

- easily losing their temper or getting annoyed
- angry and resentful behavior
- hostility toward any authoritative figure
- annoying peers

- blames others for mistakes

The overlapping symptoms can make it very hard to distinguish between ODD and ADHD, especially in younger children. Since ADHD can add fuel to the ODD fire, it's vital to diagnose both of these conditions.

ADHD and Obsessive-Compulsive Disorder

Obsessive-compulsive disorder (OCD) is a mental health condition characterized by unwanted, intrusive thoughts (obsessions) and repetitive behaviors (compulsions) (Mayo Clinic Staff, 2023). These obsessions and compulsions can be time-consuming and distressing, significantly interfering with daily life. Obsessions are recurrent, persistent, and unwanted thoughts, urges, or images that often cause anxiety or distress, and examples include the fear of contamination, thoughts of harm and violence, and excessive doubt. Individuals who are driven by obsessions are compelled to repeat behavior or mental acts. Common compulsions include cleaning and washing, checking whether something was done correctly, counting, and mental rituals.

OCD is often portrayed in media as being germaphobes or perfectionists, but it's much more complex than that. OCD affects between 1% and 3% of adults, 80% of whom had symptoms before they were 18 years old (Frye, 2024). OCD and ADHD are among the most commonly diagnosed neuropsychiatric disorders. It's estimated that 30% of adults with ADHD also have OCD (Olivardia, 2021). Despite the prevalence overlap, ADHD is often missed in patients with OCD and vice versa.

Both ADHD and OCD are associated with the frontostriatal area of the brain, which is in charge of attention-shifting, flexibility, habits, and goal-directed behavior. Due to atypical activity in this area of the brain, individuals with OCD or ADHD experience struggles with decision-making, remembering important things, planning, and switching between tasks.

ADHD and Anxiety

Anxiety is a mental health condition characterized by excessive worry, fear, and nervousness that can interfere with daily life (American Psychiatric Association, 2022). It can manifest as persistent restlessness, difficulty concentrating, muscle tension, and even physical symptoms like headaches or gastrointestinal discomfort. While ADHD and anxiety disorder are distinct conditions, they often co-occur, making diagnosis and treatment more complex.

One reason ADHD and anxiety frequently appear together is that individuals with ADHD often face chronic stress due to difficulties in organization, time management, and impulse control (Kooij et al., 2019). These struggles can lead to feelings of failure, frustration, and uncertainty, increasing anxiety levels over time. Additionally, the brain structures involved in emotional regulation, such as the prefrontal cortex and amygdala, are implicated in both conditions, further contributing to their connection (Volkow et al., 2021). There are several overlapping symptoms between ADHD and anxiety, including restlessness, difficulty focusing, and excessive worry. However, a key difference is that ADHD-related distraction is often due to inattention and external stimuli, while anxiety-driven distraction stems from internal worries (Barkley, 2020).

The combination of ADHD and anxiety can be particularly dangerous. Individuals may experience heightened emotional dysregulation, extreme procrastination, and difficulty managing responsibilities, leading to issues in work, school, and personal relationships (Pliszka, 2019). Moreover, untreated anxiety can worsen ADHD symptoms, creating a cycle of stress and impaired functioning. Understanding the connection between these conditions is essential for proper management, which may involve therapy, medication, or lifestyle changes tailored to both disorders.

ADHD and Depression

Depression is a condition characterized by persistent changes in mood or a lack of interest in daily activities (Rodden, 2023). It's quite common and affects roughly 14.8 million American adults. Women are 70% more likely to experience major depression than men, and two-thirds of all reported suicides in the U.S. are attributed to depression each year (Rodden, 2023). Yet, very few people seek proper treatment. One reason for this is that many are unaware that their experiences are symptoms of a treatable condition. Due to the overlapping symptoms of anxiety and ADHD, many are unaware of their depression. Symptoms of depression include the following (Cleveland Clinic, 2023b):

- **Persistent sadness, anxiety, or emptiness:** This is often the most noticeable symptom of depression. It's not just feeling down but a deep sense of sadness, hopelessness, and emptiness that doesn't go away.

- **Loss of interest or pleasure:** This is known as anhedonia. People with depression may lose interest in activities they once enjoyed, such as hobbies, sports, or spending time with loved ones.

- **Changes in appetite or weight:** This can manifest as

either decreased appetite and weight loss or increased appetite and weight gain.

- **Sleep difficulties:** This can include insomnia (difficulty falling asleep or staying asleep) or hypersomnia (sleeping too much).

- **Fatigue or loss of energy:** Even small tasks can feel exhausting for people with depression.

- **Feelings of worthlessness or guilt:** People with depression may feel worthless, hopeless, or guilty about things they haven't done or things they feel they've done wrong.

- **Difficulty concentrating or making decisions:** It can be hard to focus, remember things, or make even simple decisions.

- **Restlessness or irritability:** People with depression may feel agitated, restless, or irritable.

- **Thoughts of death or suicide:** In severe cases, depression can lead to suicidal thoughts or attempts.

If you have ADHD, you have a higher chance of experiencing depression as well. This can be due to the emotional rollercoaster of ADHD and struggles with emotional regulation, as well as constantly feeling like a failure and experiencing pressure to be better. According to studies, teen girls who are diagnosed between the ages of 6 and 18 are more likely to experience depression and suicidal thoughts than their peers (Roth, 2019). For many people, untreated ADHD can lead to depression due to the constant struggles, failures, and attempts to be "normal." Since ADHD can cause trouble with school, social life, and daily activities, it can make undiagnosed ADHDers feel bad about themselves, making them prone to negative self-concept (Sherman, 2019).

ADHD and Autism

Autism spectrum Disorder (ASD) is a complex neurobiological disorder that can be characterized by difficulty communicating and relating to others, as well as the need to engage in repetitive behavior and language (Rodden, 2024). Similar to ADHD, ASD occurs on a broad continuum. People with this disorder might present very differently from one another, and each patient should be treated uniquely—not with a one-size-fits-all approach. ASD affects many people. Studies have found that approximately 1 in 36 children in the U.S. has ASD, and it's four times more common in boys than girls (Rodden, 2024). Symptoms of autism include:

- finding it challenging to engage in a back-and-forth conversation

- struggling with nonverbal communication, such as eye contact, and finds it hard to read body language

- experiencing difficulties with maintaining and understanding relationships

- engaging in repetitive behavior and movements

- struggling with change and anything that doesn't fit within the routine

- engaging in specific, fixated interests

Both ADHD and ASD are neurodevelopmental disorders and impact similar brain functions, which causes an overlap in symptoms. The biggest difference between autism and ADHD is a willingness to embrace change and communication. While ADHDers often struggle to communicate deep and honest feelings due to the pressure to mask their true feelings, autistic individuals find it very difficult to communicate effectively with others. When ADHD and ASD exist in tandem, it can very often lead to a third disorder: anxiety (ADDitude Editors & Perlis,

2022). When autism and ADHD co-occur, it's often referred to as AuDHD. Although there are many similarities in autism and ADHD symptoms, there are also many differences that can be used to diagnose both these conditions.

ADHD and Sensory Processing Disorder

Sensory processing disorder (SPD) is a feeling of anxiety that occurs when you experience too much sensory input. While it can be a standalone disorder, it's a very common symptom in those with ADHD (Burch, 2024). SPD can make it very difficult to focus on everyday tasks and can cause feelings of being overwhelmed. It's often described as "overload," where it feels like everything is just too loud. This can be triggered by the simplest things, and it doesn't necessarily require a super loud environment.

A client I worked with recently experienced severe sensory overload while on a road trip. They were driving through a beautiful mountain pass with the radio playing their favorite music. As they were driving through the pass, filled with twists and turns, the aircon was blasting cool air, and they were enjoying some sour gummies—their favorite. Individually, every element of what was happening was positive: the scenery, music, snacks, and cool air. However, altogether, the changes in the car were too much, and they experienced sensory overload. The client immediately asked their husband to pull over so they could catch their breath, clear their mouth with some water, and allow their brain to cool down before continuing on the journey (this time, without music and snacks).

There are a few reasons why ADHDers are more susceptible to SPD. The first is due to a lack of self-regulation. Since those with ADHD struggle with emotional regulation, what might seem like a minor irritation to neurotypical people can result in an outburst. ADHDers also struggle with transitions, which contribute to uncomfortable situations and sensory overload. Lastly, individuals diagnosed with ADHD often lack awareness as they get distracted, disorganized, and rushed. This can lead to dealing with sensations they don't like, adding to the stress they're already experiencing.

SPD, as a standalone disorder, is often confused with ADHD. However, even though these disorders overlap, they can also exist separately from one another. There are three types of sensory disorders, including (Kranowitz, 2025):

- **Sensory over-responsivity:** This is where you will avoid certain sensory stimulations. In fact, you'll go out of your way to avoid that sensation. For example, covering your ears with your hands, closing your eyes, or hiding under the covers.

- **Sensory under-responsivity:** This type doesn't notice what's going on around them. If you have this type, you might appear withdrawn because you are unaware of the sensory stimuli around you. In other words, you're not excited about the newly painted wall because you honestly didn't notice it.

- **Sensory craving:** This type occurs when you seek sensory stimulation all the time. You want as much sensation as possible. This is often the daredevil who jumps off high bridges or who wants to go the fastest. No amount of sensory input is enough, and they always want more and more.

ADHD and Post-Traumatic Stress Disorder

Post-traumatic stress disorder (PTSD) refers to a mental health condition that develops after something deeply distressing has been experienced or witnessed. It often comes with intrusive thoughts, flashbacks, nightmares, and heightened alertness (American Psychiatric Association, 2022). While ADHD and PTSD seem like completely different disorders, they frequently show up together, making life even more challenging.

ADHDers are often at a higher risk of experiencing trauma. Impulsivity and poor risk assessment can sometimes lead to dangerous situations (Sullivan et al., 2019). At the same time, ADHD makes it harder to process emotions and cope with stress, which can increase the likelihood of developing PTSD after a traumatic event (Ford & Connor, 2020). On the flip side, PTSD can make ADHD symptoms worse or even mimic them, often leading to a misdiagnosis (Wilens et al., 2021).

There's a lot of overlap between these two conditions. Both can cause difficulty with focus, emotional ups and downs, sleep issues, and impulsivity (Kessler et al., 2018). However, the key difference is that PTSD symptoms come from trauma-related hypervigilance, whereas ADHD is rooted in brain development differences. This is why it's so important to get the right diagnosis—treating one but ignoring the other can make symptoms spiral.

When ADHD and PTSD team up, things can get tough. Emotional outbursts, risk-taking, difficulty with relationships, and even self-destructive behaviors can become major challenges (Weiss et al., 2020). Untreated PTSD can also make ADHD-related impulsivity worse, increasing the risk of substance abuse, depression, or even suicidal thoughts. That's why getting the right support—whether through therapy, medication, or trauma-informed care—is essential for managing both conditions and improving quality of life.

ADHD and Borderline Personality Disorder

Borderline personality disorder (BPD) is a mental health condition characterized by instability in relationships, emotions, and self-image (Morales, 2022). People with BPD often experience intense emotions that are hard to control. They also have a distorted sense of self, which can lead to impulsive and risky behavior. BPD is one of 10 personality disorders and isn't the only one that can coexist with ADHD. However, it is one of the most common personality disorders to act in tandem with ADHD, as 10% of ADHDers are also diagnosed with BPD. Symptoms of BPD include the following (Morales, 2022):

- **Unstable moods:** People with BPD often experience intense and rapid mood swings, sometimes shifting from extreme happiness to deep sadness or anger within hours or even minutes.

- **Unstable relationships:** People with BPD may have difficulty maintaining healthy relationships due to their intense emotions and fear of abandonment. They may idealize others at first but then quickly devalue them if they feel let down or rejected.

- **Distorted sense of self:** People with BPD may have a fluctuating and unstable sense of self, including their identity, goals, and values. This can lead to feelings of emptiness and confusion about who they are.

- **Impulsive and risky behaviors:** BPD can lead to impulsive and risky behaviors like substance abuse, reckless driving, gambling, or self-harm. This symptom overlaps with ADHD, making it hard to diagnose within ADHDers.

- **Fear of abandonment:** People with BPD often have an intense fear of being abandoned or rejected, which can lead to desperate efforts to avoid being alone.

- **Self-harm:** People with BPD may engage in self-harm behaviors, such as cutting, burning, or picking at their skin, as a way to cope with emotional distress. They may also experience suicidal thoughts or attempt suicide.

BPD and ADHD can share similar attributes, which can make it hard to distinguish one from the other. While individuals with ADHD experience wild emotional rides, they have a clear sense of who they are and their goals. They might get frustrated by their goals and their failed attempts, but they don't usually lose track of themselves. Other signs of BPD that don't overlap with ADHD include self-sabotaging behavior, brief psychotic symptoms, and the fear of abandonment by others (Morales, 2022).

With all of these disorders, kindness and acceptance are extremely important. Getting a diagnosis doesn't mean doom and gloom. These disorders are treatable, and you don't have to suffer in silence for the rest of your life. If you resonate deeply with any of these disorders we've discussed, I highly suggest you speak to your healthcare provider about it. Remember to advocate for yourself! Unfortunately, many healthcare providers are hesitant to dig deep and find the right diagnosis. So, if you're unhappy with your care, don't be scared to seek a second (or third) opinion.

Now that we've covered the foundations of ADHD, it's time to look at some practical management strategies. In the next chapter, we'll focus specifically on strategies for children and teens. So, if you're a parent or caretaker of an ADHD child or

teen, be sure to embrace these management techniques to help
the ADHDer in your life.

Chapter 5:

Management Strategies for Children and Teens

ADHD is not a choice or bad parenting. Kids with ADHD work twice as hard as their peers every day but receive more negative feedback from the world. -DRB

Watching your child struggle with ADHD can be heartbreaking. I've met so many parents filled with desperation, sadness, guilt, and even anger. One mother I spoke with recently made the following remark: "I know he doesn't do it on purpose, so why do I still get so mad?" While she felt completely alone, her question was far more common than she thought. In fact, many parents or caretakers of those diagnosed with ADHD experience this frustration. It's okay to get frustrated and even angry sometimes. You're only a human trying to do your best, but unfortunately, there is no life manual for this world to help us troubleshoot our struggles. So, don't be so hard on yourself. The important thing is that you're trying to help and support the ADHDer in your life.

I'm sure you've also experienced your fair share of judgment from others and perhaps even yourself, so let me remind you that ADHD isn't due to poor parenting. It's not your fault that this is something your child is struggling with. One of the biggest frustrations with parenting an ADHDer occurs when parents use neurotypical parenting tools and styles to parent their neurodivergent child. Just as neurodivergent adults need specific tools to help them with daily tasks, ADHD children respond differently to parenting techniques than neurotypical children. However, even when you're frustrated, don't view ADHD as the enemy. In doing so, it will only create a subconscious wedge between you and your ADHDer.

As we look at some techniques to help parent your ADHDer, I want to preface it all by saying there's no one right way to parent. As a parent, you know your child better than I do—use that to your advantage. Don't dismiss any advice or tools that you may feel won't work, but also don't waste time on methods that you've tried and didn't work. Be open to adapting and customizing each tool and technique to specifically fit your child's needs. The goal of this chapter is not to judge your parenting or all the methods you've tried in the past. It's to equip and empower you for the way ahead, making your life easier while ensuring your child receives the necessary support.

Setting the Rules

The first step to finding parenting techniques and tools to help your ADHDer is to determine what is acceptable and what isn't. What does that look like? It starts with identifying what the core values of your family are. This part of the process isn't about setting every small rule you have but rather identifying the heart of what is or is not acceptable within the family values. For example, core values might be honesty and transparency. You will then use these core values to determine the course of action going forward.

Let's put it into practice: One of the biggest problems parents have with their ADHD children is that they may not make their bed every morning. Many parents are concerned that this is a sign of poor hygiene or a lack of care. The truth is, most ADHDers just don't realize their bed isn't made because they have to use all their energy to get out of bed and get dressed (and remember to do the thousand other things that come naturally to neurotypicals). So, what can you do about it? Ask yourself—is making the bed a core value in your family? Probably not, right? In the grand scheme of things, making the bed is a small thing. In fact, it's not just ADHDers who struggle with this task. Many neurotypicals struggle to make their bed. Some rules in your home might need to be adapted for ADHD, while others simply reflect adolescent behavior.

Once you've identified your core values, you can use them to create new rules for your child. For example, they may struggle with making their bed but really enjoy feeding the dogs because it provides them with interaction and excitement. If teamwork is one of your core values, why not combine these options and create a balanced morning routine? For example, instead of your ADHDer making their bed before school and your neurotypical child feeding the dogs, they could swap chores and tackle them as a team.

It's vital not to sweat the small stuff but to create workarounds that still align with your family's core values. Another example might be if your child doesn't want to eat their lunch at the table. It's a core value that everyone should be nourished, but it's not important if your child doesn't sit at the table every lunch. Ask yourself, is it more important that my child eat or that he sits still at the table and eats? While it might sound unconventional, it's okay for your child to take his lunch outside and eat on the swing set or sit underneath the table and pretend to camp. The key is to evaluate why certain "traditional" rules are in place. If it's simply a rule to make everything feel or seem more "normal," then perhaps it shouldn't be a rule in your home at all.

Consistency, Clarity, and Negotiations

Giving your ADHD child more room to negotiate rules doesn't mean letting them call the shots. However, it does remove some of the rigid rules, allowing you and your child to work together to find new ways to accommodate one another. The success of this depends on clarity and open communication. Everyone in the household should be aware of the family's rules and values. They should know that in your house, you value teamwork, kindness, laughter, honesty, and trying your best. Keep the rules simple, but remind your family of them frequently. When your child's behavior doesn't align with these rules, gently remind them and be consistent with consequences. By approaching your day this way—rather than enforcing strict rules and rigid schedules—you give your child the freedom they need to thrive with their ADHD.

Another important element is to encourage open discussions for negotiations while being firm with strict boundaries. Your family values shouldn't be up for negotiation, but other rules can be flexible. If this sounds crazy right now, give it a chance. Remember, negotiating means that you work together to find a solution that works for you both. For example, let's say it's time to do homework, but your ADHDer is really struggling to focus because she just saw that a new episode of her favorite show is out. All she can think of is the show, no matter how hard she tries. So, instead of creating frustration for both of you, why not negotiate? Perhaps it's okay if she takes 30 minutes to watch her show before she does her homework if she also helps you in the kitchen after dinner. The rules that are up for negotiation don't have to be connected to one another as long as they align with your family values. Will her homework get done? Yes, just later than usual. Will she embrace teamwork because you have? Absolutely.

Tools for Managing Emotions

Emotional management is something every child needs to learn. We're not born with the ability to self-regulate and manage our emotions effectively. Instead, we're born with an inherent desire to act on our emotions as that's how we get our needs taken care of. Babies cry to signal that they need care, yet, somewhere along the line, we expect children should just *know* how to do this effectively. ADHD children especially struggle to acquire this skill, and they need extra guidance to learn it. ADHDers experience intense emotions, which can cause them to feel overwhelmed quickly. One moment, they might be having the best day of their lives, and the next, they're crashing and hating everything. They also have trouble identifying what they're feeling, so they might feel upset but they might not be aware of why. Is it fear? Stress? Disappointment? They struggle more than neurotypical children to understand the differences between these emotions.

ADHD children are also more impulsive, which means managing emotions often gets placed on the back burner. They often act before they speak, which can lead to conflict and breaking the rules. While not all children with ADHD experience emotional dysregulation in the same way, there are some general tools that you can use that will help your child with this. Here is one of the best tools you can implement with your ADHDer.

Labeling Feelings

Since ADHDers struggle to identify what they are feeling, you can provide your child with additional support in this area. Labeling feelings (zones of regulation) is a technique that involves helping your child identify and name what they are experiencing. There are many other tools we can use to make this interactive, easy to understand, and more engaging for your child. For example, print out a poster with emojis on it, along with a label of what emotion they are feeling. Place the poster where they can see it and walk them through what each one means. Then, when they feel emotional, ask them to choose which one of the emojis represents what they are experiencing and name it out loud. If they point to the red-faced emoji, you can say, "Are you feeling angry? What are you angry about?" Here are a few things to keep in mind as you embrace this technique.

- **Start early:** You can begin labeling feelings with your child when they are still very young. This can also be helpful for neurotypical children, so don't restrict it to your ADHDer. Labeling emotions will help all your children develop a vocabulary for emotions and to understand that emotions are a normal part of life.

- **Use simple language:** When labeling feelings, use simple language that your child can understand. For example, you might say, "I think you're feeling angry because you're hitting the table."

- **Be specific:** Instead of saying, "You're feeling bad," try to be more specific about the emotion your child is experiencing. For example, you might say, "Are you feeling frustrated because you can't find your toy?"

- **Validate your child's feelings:** Let your child know that it's okay to feel the way they are feeling. For example, you might say, "It's okay to feel angry when you're frustrated."

- **Identify the physical sensations of different emotions:** For example, you might say, "When you're feeling sad, do you feel like crying? Do you feel like your stomach hurts?" This will help them identify the emotions themselves in the future as they begin to recognize and become aware of physical sensations.

To get started on this technique, here's a list of emotions you might want to consider adding to your visual aid to help your ADHDer identify what they are feeling. Start with only the words in bold since they are easier to identify. However, as they get older and require more variety, add some of the sub-emotions as well.

- **Happy:** joy, delight, cheerfulness, contentment, excitement, and enthusiasm
- **Love:** affection, caring, tenderness, and warmth
- **Calm:** peaceful, relaxed, serene, and comfortable
- **Proud:** confident, accomplished, and self-assured
- **Interest:** curiosity, fascination, and eagerness to learn
- **Sad:** unhappy, depressed, disappointed, and lonely
- **Angry:** mad, frustrated, irritated, and furious
- **Fear:** scared, anxious, worried, and nervous
- **Disgust:** repulsed, grossed out, and appalled
- **Surprise:** shocked, startled, and amazed

It's also important to know that not all emotions need to be discussed in the moment as this might cause more overwhelm for ADHDers. Instead, allow your child to take a second and find regulation. Then, once the worst is over, take a moment to debrief with them. During the debrief, you can discuss what happened, provide validation, and help them to improve their awareness of the situation. Simple and clear communication will show them how to identify their emotions and the situation by themselves in the future.

Structure and Routine

Structure and routine are a bit of a conundrum for ADHDers. On the one hand, they really need structure and routine to thrive. On the other hand, they hate it and need constant novelty and flexibility. As parents, you shouldn't throw out all sense of a routine but instead adopt a routine that provides some wiggle room. For example, instead of saying that homework needs to happen immediately after school, you can mention that homework needs to happen before dinner. Routine is important because it reduces decision fatigue, improves focus, and can increase productivity. But a routine that is too rigid will put more pressure on your child, and they'll be less likely to actually accomplish what they need to. Rigid adherence to a strict schedule can be stifling and can lead to feelings of frustration and resentment. The key lies in experimenting with what works for you and your child.

Steps to Creating a Routine That Works

To create a routine that works for the ADHD mind, you need to be willing to adopt flexibility, creativity, and a reward system. To help your ADHDers from feeling overwhelmed, break their daily routine into different bite sizes. For example, instead of one big routine, break the day into morning, afternoon, evening, and nighttime routines. This helps them feel more comfortable with each part, giving a sense of accomplishment after completing each section of the routine. It also helps to remove the pressure of keeping track of many things at once.

A traditional routine will usually have a list of tasks to be completed in a specific order, with precise time slots allocated to each. However, this is too rigid for your ADHDer, and the moment they lose track of time, they'll feel defeated and give up. A rigid routine will quickly become boring after a couple of days. Instead, give your ADHDer a visible list of tasks and let them decide the order in which they complete them. If they want to brush their teeth before they feed the dog, it really doesn't matter as long as everything gets done.

A big part of what makes this type of routine successful is setting up rewards for each stage. If they can physically "tick" the boxes as they're moving along with their chores, they are more likely to experience a dopamine boost and improve their productivity.

Also, if they know that there is an actual reward for accomplishing all their tasks, they will be more eager to do them. For example, if your ADHDer accomplishes all of their morning tasks before school (in whatever order they prefer), they can choose the pizza toppings for dinner or what music you'll listen to in the car on the way to school.

You can also apply these two principles to the other routines in the day. For example, instead of having a set bedtime, allow them to go to bed anywhere between 7 p.m. and 9 p.m. Or if they do all their "chores" that are part of the nighttime routine, they don't have to make their bed the next morning (or whatever other reward would inspire them). It's also important to mix things up every now and again and change the order in which you present the tasks they need to accomplish or add a fun element to the routine. For example, make their morning routine include something that they need to pull a face in the mirror or tell a joke on the way to school. These small novelties will make a big difference in how they perceive the routine and how well they respond to it.

Breaking Down Larger Tasks

Have you ever heard the joke, "How do you eat an elephant? Piece by piece." Well, breaking down tasks for your ADHDer works the same way. If they focus on the entire elephant, it can be overwhelming. Instead of getting excited, your ADHDer may only see the enormity of the task and how it feels impossible to tackle. But when you present them with one piece at a time, they'll manage it much easier and more confidently. Breaking down tasks into smaller, more manageable steps has many benefits for your ADHDer, including the following:

- **Reduces anxiety and overwhelm:** When faced with a large task, it can be difficult to know where to start, which can lead to feelings of anxiety and avoidance. By breaking the task down into smaller steps, it becomes more manageable and less daunting.

- **Improves focus and concentration:** When your ADHDer is focused on a specific, smaller task, it becomes easier for them to stay on track and avoid distractions. This is because the smaller task requires less mental effort and can be completed more quickly.

- **Increases motivation and a sense of accomplishment:** When your ADHDer can see the progress they're making on a task, it motivates them to keep going. This is especially true when the smaller steps are slightly challenging but achievable.

- **Teaches organization and planning:** By breaking down tasks into smaller steps, your ADHD child will learn how to plan and organize their work. This is a valuable skill that can be used in many areas of life, allowing them to learn powerful tools to become more independent.

To practically break down a big task into smaller bites might be challenging at first, especially if you are neurodiverse, but the idea is not to "dumb it down." Your child's problem isn't their intelligence— it's being overwhelmed and distracted when faced with a lot of information at the same time. For example, let's say they have a big presentation coming up at school and they read the instructions provided by the teacher: a long paragraph with many steps and requirements. Immediately, your ADHDer will feel overwhelmed and would literally do anything other than work on the project. Why? Because it feels impossible. Here's how you can practically help them in this scenario:

- **Step 1:** Work with your child to identify the overall goal of the task. What does the teacher want from them? A presentation on a role model.

- **Step 2:** Break down the overall goal into smaller pieces. The project requires research, a visual presentation, and a speech. Immediately, the overall project was split into three smaller tasks.

- **Step 3:** Break the three tasks into even smaller, actionable steps. Before your child can do research, they need to choose what they want to do the presentation about. They will also need to find information about the person's childhood, career, and what makes them a good role model. Write these steps down in a clear and concise manner, breaking down all the tasks into their simplest form.

- **Step 4:** Work with your child to estimate the time each step might take and set deadlines for each step. This will reduce stress later on in the journey, especially when you use a timer for each step.

- **Step 5:** Encourage your child to take breaks between steps and reward them for completing each step.

Breaking the tasks into smaller bits should be collaborative. Invite your child to work with you so they learn the skill themselves, allowing them to implement it on their own when they get older. The clearer and concise each step of the journey is, the more likely the chances of success. If your child gets overwhelmed quickly, try to reduce the information provided in one setting to help them process one thing at a time.

Limiting Distractions

Distractions look different for different people. Most neurotypicals view distractions as things that physically disrupt you from your work. For example, a colleague comes to your desk to talk to you. However, for an ADHDer, distractions can often show up in the most unexpected ways. ADHD children, in particular, might find birds outside the classroom window as a distraction, or the teacher's bouncing hairstyle can disrupt their train of thought. As a parent, you can help limit these distractions. You should know that your child isn't getting distracted on purpose or just to annoy you. They can't help that their pencil looks like a rocket ship. However, even though they can't help it, there are some practical things you and your child can do together to ensure distractions are limited.

Limiting Distractions at Home

There are many things that can distract your ADHDer at home, especially when they need to focus on a specific task (or a simple conversation). While it's impossible to eliminate all distractions without removing all the fun and joy from the home, there are a few simple things you can do to support your child with ADHD. Be warned, they might not enjoy the idea of these limitations at first, but it will greatly help them to concentrate. And as soon as they experience the benefits, they are more likely to be open to these and similar changes. Here are a few ideas you can implement:

- **Designated workspace:** Designate a specific area for studying or homework that is free from clutter and distractions. Ensure that this space has good lighting and minimal noise. Even decor should be approached with a more minimalistic style to create a calm and focused environment.

- **Technology rules:** When it's time to focus, be sure to turn off the TV, radio, and phones. You can also consider investing in noise-canceling headphones or a white noise machine. If you have more than one child with ADHD, it might be helpful to align their focus times to avoid each ADHDer getting distracted by the other child's entertainment. Even if the television is on the opposite side of the house, your ADHDer might hear some noise and experience FOMO, making it even harder to focus.

- **Visual timers and schedules:** Use visual schedules or timers to break down tasks and manage time. This will help your ADHDer to see the end goal and stay on track.

Limiting Distractions at School

You can't control your child's school environment all the time, which can be a scary thought. ADHDers can experience a lot of distractions in a classroom as most school systems do not take into account the needs of ADHDers. As a parent, you can support your child at school by doing the following:

- **Communicate with the teacher:** Work closely with teachers to ensure that you both understand your child's specific needs and challenges. You can also discuss potential classroom adjustments with the teacher, such as seating arrangements, preferential seating, and additional chores during the day to help them physically.

- **Organization tools:** Your child will most likely struggle to stay on top of things. For example, they might forget about permission slips and homework. You can help them from a young age by putting certain tools in place. For example, have a designated "dump" place where every day after school, they completely empty their backpack into a container (without any judgment from anyone). No matter if the papers are crumpled up or the lunch half-eaten—it's a safe space for them to just dump the day. Later, you and your child can look through the dumped contents together and create a system to help them at school be prepared and organized.. What can go in the bin? What is homework or important notes? What belongs to a friend and needs to be sent back?

- **Teach self-regulation:** The best way to help your child is to equip them so they can eventually help themselves. One way to do this is by teaching them self-regulation methods. This can include strategies such as deep breathing, thinking out loud, and wait time strategy. The wait time strategy involves teaching your ADHDer to tolerate brief periods of unstructured time or waiting. By practicing waiting, they can improve their ability to focus and resist distractions.

Helping your child to manage their ADHD isn't a one-size-fits-all approach. You and your child will have to work together, in collaboration with educators and possibly other professionals, to find specific tools and techniques that work for your child's unique needs. As important as it is for children to grow and learn to manage their ADHD, it's equally important for adults with ADHD to do the same. In the next chapter, we'll look at a few ADHD-friendly tools and techniques that every ADHD adult should implement in their daily life to improve symptom management.

Chapter 6:

ADHD Management Strategies for Adults

My mind is like my web browser: 19 tabs are open, 3 are frozen, and I have no idea where the music is coming from. –Anonymous

I love this quote, and I often use it in my practice. While it's funny and lighthearted, it actually perfectly covers the real issues and experiences of an ADHDer. When you have so many tabs open in your mind, it's very hard to maneuver around them. It's almost like you get stuck on these different pages, and you have to use all your energy to get to the one you're actually looking for. During this process, you're trying to feed your mind even more information while trying to guide it back to the page you're looking for. This ultimately leads to your browser lagging and struggling to keep track of everything, and in turn, you'll become frustrated, anxious, and just give up.

As an adult with ADHD, you experience many situations like this on a daily basis, which is why it's so important to learn the right strategies to manage your symptoms. Chances are, you've tried numerous techniques before with very little success. Why? Because most techniques, tools, and strategies are too generic as they are created for neurotypical minds. In this chapter, we'll look at what makes a strategy ADHD-friendly and how you can adapt different tools to ensure it works for you. We'll look at tools for organization and time management, communication and relationships, and emotional management. But first, let's take a look at the two non-negotiables of every ADHD-friendly strategy.

The Two Non-Negotiables of Every ADHD Strategy

When it comes to the difference between ADHD and neurotypical strategies and neurotypical, there are two factors that continuously play a role: flexibility and creativity. These two elements are the pillars of a successful ADHD strategy as they provide the ADHD brain with all it needs. Their importance stems from the very nature of ADHD, which often presents unique challenges and requires personalized approaches. Let's take a closer look at what they both mean and how you can implement them.

Flexibility

When it comes to ADHD strategies, flexibility is paramount. Rigid routines and inflexible expectations can quickly become obstacles for ADHDers. Life with ADHD is often unpredictable, with fluctuating energy levels, shifting interests, and unexpected distractions. A more strict approach can lead to frustration, burnout, and a sense of failure. Instead, flexible strategies allow for adjustments based on your needs and circumstances. This might involve modifying schedules, adapting to changing priorities, or finding alternative ways to accomplish goals. For example, if a planned study session is disrupted by a sudden burst of energy, a flexible approach might involve incorporating a quick physical activity before returning to the task. Here are a few examples of how you can embrace flexibility:

- **Adjusting schedules:** If your morning routine is consistently thrown off by a late start, be flexible and adjust your schedule accordingly. Instead of rigidly adhering to a timetable, prioritize key activities and allow for flexibility in their timing.

- **Adapting to changes:** Unexpected events are common. If a meeting runs longer than expected, be flexible and adjust your subsequent plans. Don't get bogged down by the disruption; instead, find a way to make it work.

- **Openness to new ideas:** Be open to new ways of doing things, even if they deviate from your usual routine. This could involve trying a different route to work, exploring a new hobby, or adopting a new organizational system.

Creativity

Creativity is equally valuable, as it empowers ADHDers to find unique solutions to their challenges. The ADHD brain often possesses strengths in divergent thinking, allowing for innovative problem-solving and the ability to see connections others might miss. Encouraging creativity in ADHD strategies can involve exploring different approaches to tasks, finding unique ways to stay organized, and harnessing strengths to compensate for weaknesses. For instance, you might find it challenging to maintain focus during traditional meetings. A creative solution could involve recording the meeting and listening to it later at your own pace, allowing for pausing and rewinding as needed.

Even when you consider yourself imaginative, the ADHD brain craves the novelty that creativity provides. Being creative doesn't necessarily mean you are proficient in arts and crafts. Instead, it means you embrace an alternative approach to getting things done that is different from what is considered traditional and "normal." Here are a few examples of what embracing creativity might look like:

- **Finding unique solutions:** When faced with a challenge, think outside the box. Instead of resorting to conventional solutions, brainstorm creative approaches that may be more effective or enjoyable for you.

- **Harnessing strengths:** Identify your strengths and find ways to leverage them in your daily life. If you're a creative person, find ways to incorporate that creativity into your work or hobbies. If you thrive on multitasking, use that to your advantage in managing household tasks.

- **Experimenting with techniques:** Experiment with different techniques for managing your time, staying organized, or improving your focus. This could involve trying different productivity apps, using visual reminders, or incorporating movement breaks into your routine.

With these two pillars in mind, we can now approach specific management tools and apply these principles to each to ensure that we adopt tools that are actually ADHD-friendly.

Organization and Time Management Tools

Organization and time management can be significant hurdles for ADHDers due to challenges with focus, impulsivity, and difficulties prioritizing tasks. However, by implementing effective strategies and utilizing available tools, you can gain greater control over your time, improve your productivity, and reduce feelings of being overwhelmed. Let's take a closer look at some tools that will empower you to enhance your efficiency, reduce stress, and achieve your goals.

Timeboxing

What it is: Timeboxing is a powerful technique for ADHD adults because it provides a structured framework that counteracts the inherent challenges of ADHD, such as impulsivity, procrastination, and difficulty with time perception. However, when set up correctly, it's not too linear or rigid.

How it works: Allocate specific blocks of time for different activities, even when they are short. Use that specific time block to work on the task at hand, but grant yourself the freedom to do it in whatever order you'd like.

The benefits: The benefits of timeboxing for ADHDers are numerous. Firstly, it helps to combat procrastination. By setting specific time limits for tasks, timeboxing creates a sense of urgency and can help break down large, overwhelming projects into smaller, more manageable chunks. This can be particularly helpful for tasks that are perceived as boring or difficult. Timeboxing also helps to improve focus. When you know you only have a limited amount of time to work on a task, it can help you stay on track and minimize distractions. This is because you're less likely to get sidetracked by other thoughts or activities if you're aware that your time is limited. Thirdly, timeboxing helps to reduce anxiety. The fear of not completing tasks can be a significant source of anxiety for any ADHDer, and alleviating this anxiety by providing a clear structure and a sense of control over your time.

How to personalize it: The best tools and strategies are those you can personalize and make your own. By experimenting with the time intervals, you can create your own timeboxing system. Find intervals that work for you, whether that's longer or shorter than suggested by the others. You can also adjust the intervals based on day-to-day tasks and circumstances. When you're experiencing a bad day, you can make the intervals shorter, while during hyperfocus, you can make them longer.

Prioritization Techniques

What it is: Prioritization techniques are methods for determining the order in which you tackle tasks, ensuring you focus on the most important ones first. This helps combat the tendency to get sidetracked by less critical or more appealing activities. There are various types of prioritization techniques that you can use, including the Eisenhower Matrix, the Pareto Principle, and the ABCDE method.

How it works: Begin by listing all the tasks you need to accomplish. This could include work projects, errands, household chores, personal goals, etc. Depending on the technique you're using, you can then follow the steps to prioritize your day. As an example, the Eisenhower Matrix categorizes tasks into four quadrants:

1. Urgent and important (do these tasks first)

2. Important but not urgent (these are tasks you can schedule for later)

3. Urgent but not important (these tasks can be delegated to someone else)

4. Neither urgent nor important (these tasks should be eliminated as they are time-wasters and distractions)

The benefits: Prioritization techniques reduce overwhelm by providing you with a sense of control. It also increases your productivity as it helps you to focus on important tasks first. This naturally also improves focus and reduces procrastination. When you know which tasks are most critical, you are less likely to waste time on tasks that should actually be eliminated or delegated.

How to personalize it: You can personalize prioritization techniques by using visual aids like mind maps and color-coding to make it more tangible. You can also make it your own by experimenting with different methods and perhaps combining two traditional methods to create one that works for you. Remember to be flexible. Life is dynamic, and your priorities will change. It's okay to move tasks from one quadrant to another.

Visual Aids

What it is: Visual aids are tools that use visual cues to enhance organization, memory, and focus. For ADHDers, these aids can be incredibly valuable in overcoming challenges related to attention, impulsivity, and time management.

How it works: Visual aids bypass the limitations of working memory, which can be impaired in individuals with ADHD. By presenting information visually, these aids reduce the cognitive load and make it easier to process and retain information. Visual tools like calendars, to-do lists, and mind maps also help to organize thoughts, tasks, and schedules in a clear and concise manner.

The benefits: Visual aids can help to enhance focus by directing attention and minimizing distractions, making it easier to stay on task and on track. It can also improve memory by triggering associations, making it easier to recall information and complete tasks. Additionally, visual aids also increase organization and time management as they can help you to reduce any feelings of overwhelm and the temptation to procrastinate.

How to personalize it: The best way to personalize visual aids is to experiment with different types of aids, such as calendars, mind maps, habit trackers, etc., to see what works best for you. You can also incorporate color and imagery into your visual aids to make them more engaging and memorable. For example, use colored pens to highlight important information or use images to represent different tasks. The best part of visual aids is making them fun. For example, use stickers, decorative tape, or any other fun future to add a personal touch. By experimenting with different visual aids and finding what works best for you, you can harness the power of visual learning to improve your organization, focus, and overall productivity.

Auditory Cues

What it is: Auditory tools use sound-based cues to support focus, memory, and emotional regulation. For ADHDers, these tools can be incredibly helpful in overcoming challenges related to attention, task initiation, and sensory processing.

How it works: Auditory tools tap into the brain's ability to process sound in ways that enhance focus and reduce distractions. Since many individuals with ADHD struggle with executive function and working memory, auditory cues can serve as external reminders that keep them engaged and on track. Background sounds, verbal prompts, or rhythmic cues help structure time and provide motivation. Examples of auditory tools include white noise machines, guided meditations, audiobooks, timers, and text-to-speech programs.

The benefits: Auditory tools can improve focus by minimizing distractions and creating a structured auditory environment. White noise, instrumental music, or nature sounds can help ADHDers filter out background noise and sustain attention on tasks. Verbal reminders and alarms assist with memory by providing real-time prompts for tasks and deadlines. Additionally, auditory tools support emotional regulation by offering soothing sounds or guided relaxation exercises to manage stress and overwhelm.

How to personalize it: The key to making auditory tools effective is experimenting with different types of sounds and cues. Some people find that instrumental music helps them concentrate, while others prefer nature sounds or binaural beats.

Smart speakers and apps can be programmed to provide verbal reminders while using a metronome, or rhythmic beats can help with time management and task pacing. Audiobooks and podcasts can make learning more engaging for those who absorb information better through listening. The best part? You can mix and match different tools to create an environment that keeps you focused and motivated in a way that feels natural to you.

Communication and Relationship Tools

Effective communication is a must for building healthy relationships, but it can pose unique challenges for ADHDers. Difficulties with focus, impulsivity, and emotional regulation can sometimes lead to misunderstandings, conflicts, and strained relationships. However, employing specific strategies and utilizing available tools can help you significantly improve your communication skills. Here are three tools you can use to navigate the complexities of interpersonal relationships with greater ease and confidence.

Active Listening

What it is: Active listening is a communication technique that goes beyond simply hearing the words spoken by another person. It involves paying close attention to both verbal and nonverbal cues, demonstrating genuine interest and empathy, and providing feedback to ensure understanding.

How it works: Active listening consists of various elements that you can incorporate into every conversation. The best part is that you can adopt these elements one at a time (bite-size). If the idea of changing your communication completely feels overwhelming, focus on one of the following at a time until you feel comfortable enough to add another.

- **Focus on the speaker:** Give the speaker your undivided attention. Minimize distractions like your phone, the television, or other people.

- **Maintain eye contact:** Maintain eye contact with the speaker, but avoid staring intensely.

- **Observe body language:** Pay attention to the speaker's body language, including their posture, gestures, and facial expressions. These nonverbal cues often convey more information than words alone.

- **Listen to the tone of voice:** Take note of the speaker's tone of voice. It can indicate their emotions, such as anger, sadness, or excitement.

- **Paraphrase:** Briefly summarize what you've heard to ensure you've understood correctly. For example, "So, it sounds like you're saying..."

- **Check for accuracy:** Ask the speaker if your summary is accurate. "Is that correct?" or "Did I understand that correctly?"

- **Acknowledge feelings:** Acknowledge and validate the speaker's feelings, even if you don't agree with them. For example, "I can understand why you feel that way."

- **Avoid interruptions:** Allow the speaker to finish their thoughts before asking questions. Even if you're excited or scared, you'll forget what you wanted to say.

The benefits: Active listening helps to reduce misunderstandings that can arise from distractions or difficulties in processing information. By demonstrating genuine interest and empathy, active listening strengthens relationships and builds trust. Carefully listening to others' perspectives helps to prevent conflicts that may arise from misinterpretations or assumptions. Active listening also increases self-awareness, allowing you to gain insight into your communication styles and areas for improvement.

How to personalize it: To personalize this technique, start small. Choose one or two elements to focus on so as not to overwhelm yourself. Also, begin by practicing active listening in casual, low-pressure conversations. You can also personalize it by creating a mnemonic device to help you remember the key components of active listening (e.g., "L.I.S.T.E.N." - Listen, Inquire, Summarize, Tune in, Empathize, Note). Lastly, reflect on which techniques worked for you and had a positive effect by asking a trusted friend or family member for feedback on your listening skills.

Scheduled Check-Ins

What it is: Scheduled check-ins are dedicated time slots specifically set aside for communication and connection within a relationship. These check-ins can be brief daily conversations or longer weekly or bi-weekly discussions, depending on the needs and preferences of the individuals involved.

How it works: Schedule a time slot each week to check in with friends and family to ensure that you stay in touch and don't drift apart. This will also allow for a deeper connection, showing your friends that you care for them. The consistency of a regular check-in creates a predictable routine, making it easier to remember and prioritize communication.

The benefits: Regular communication can help to prevent misunderstandings and address issues before they escalate into major conflicts. By prioritizing open and honest communication, scheduled check-ins can strengthen bonds and deepen intimacy. These dedicated conversations can create space for deeper connections, allowing you to share your thoughts, feelings, and experiences more openly. Additionally, regular check-ins also provide an opportunity for emotional support and encouragement for both you and the person you're checking in with.

How to personalize it: You can personalize this technique by choosing how often you want to have check-ins, as well as how formal the check-ins should be. One week, you might want to give them a call, and the following week, you might feel like messaging them instead. The important thing is that you find a consistent routine that works for you and the other person.

Communication Apps

What it is: The purpose of communication apps is to facilitate communication and collaboration between individuals. They offer a variety of features, such as instant messaging, video conferencing, file sharing, and more.

How it works: Communication apps allow for real-time text-based communication, enabling quick and easy exchange of messages, thoughts, and reminders. Many of these communication apps also offer features for scheduling appointments and setting reminders for events, making it easy to schedule check-ins with others. Some apps also enable face-to-face communication through video calls, which can be helpful for maintaining connections and building rapport. All that is required from you is to download the app and create a profile.

The benefits: One of the biggest benefits of communication apps for ADHDers is that they provide readily accessible platforms for quick and easy communication. This can improve communication and remove the reliance on memory when it comes to communicating with others. Communication apps can also enhance organization with features such as shared calendars, to-do lists, and other reminders, in turn reducing frustration. It also allows space and time to clarify when there's been a misunderstanding, and it keeps track of the conversation, allowing you to go back and revisit the important points. Lastly, communication apps also offer flexibility. Some days, you might want to have a face-to-face talk with someone, but on days when you feel overwhelmed, you might rather just send a message and wait for their response.

How to personalize it: You can personalize using communication apps in various ways to ensure that it works for you and doesn't add to the stress or possibility of miscommunication. Here are a few ideas:

- **Choose the right apps:** Explore different communication apps and choose those that best suit your needs and preferences. Consider factors like ease of use, features, and compatibility with your devices.

- **Establish communication guidelines:** Discuss and agree upon communication guidelines, such as response times, appropriate communication channels, and how to handle sensitive topics.

- **Minimize distractions:** Set boundaries and minimize distractions during communication, such as turning off notifications from other apps or designating specific times for checking messages.

- **Utilize features effectively:** Explore and utilize the various features offered by the chosen apps to maximize their benefits for your relationship.

- **Regularly review and adjust:** Regularly review your communication habits and adjust your use of communication apps as needed to ensure they continue to support your relationship effectively.

Emotional Management Tools

We know by now that emotional regulation can be a significant challenge for ADHDers due to factors such as impulsivity, difficulty with emotional recognition, and heightened emotional reactivity. There are various strategies and tools that can be effectively employed to enhance emotional awareness, manage emotional responses, and cultivate greater emotional stability. Let's take a look at a few management tools that will equip you with the necessary skills to navigate your emotional landscape with greater ease and resilience.

Mindfulness Techniques

What it is: By practicing mindfulness, you intentionally focus on the present moment without judging it. It involves cultivating awareness of thoughts, feelings, sensations, and the surrounding environment (Mayo Clinic Staff, 2022).

How it works: Mindfulness allows you to shift your focus away from racing thoughts and worries about the past and the future and bring your attention to the present moment. In doing so, it increases your self-awareness, allowing you to observe your thoughts and feelings without judgment. This allows you to become more aware of your emotional state and triggers. Additionally, mindfulness works by regulating your emotions, allowing you to pause and observe instead of acting impulsively (Mayo Clinic Staff, 2022).

The benefits: All people can benefit from mindfulness, not just ADHDers. However, it's especially helpful for adults with as it improves focus and attention. It can also reduce impulsivity as it teaches you to pause and reflect instead of reacting immediately to every situation. Mindfulness is also beneficial because it reduces stress and can help you to overcome your overwhelming feelings. In doing so, it regulates your emotions, reducing the impact of emotional outbursts.

How to personalize it: There are many mindfulness techniques, including deep breathing, grounding, and journaling. You can personalize each by experimenting with different techniques to find what resonates with you most. If your mind feels too busy, you can also make use of guided meditation or other apps that can gamify the process of mindfulness. One of the best things about mindfulness is that you can choose the length of each mindfulness activity. You don't have to meditate for hours to see results. Start with three minutes and see how it goes from there. Start small and increase the duration as you become more comfortable and find it helpful. You can also incorporate mindfulness while you're busy with other tasks. For example, you can practice deep breathing while you're driving or listen to a meditation while doing the dishes. As long as you're patient with yourself, you can customize mindfulness to fit your exact needs.

Emotional Regulation Training Skills

What it is: Emotional regulation training skills (ERTS) is a structured approach that teaches individuals specific skills to identify, understand, and manage their emotions. It's designed to help individuals develop greater awareness of their emotional states, recognize the triggers that lead to emotional dysregulation, and learn effective coping strategies to manage their emotions in a healthy way (Fresco et al., 2013).

How it works: ERTS typically involves a combination of psychoeducation, cognitive restructuring, relaxation techniques, and problem-solving strategies. Here's a closer look at what each of these means:

- **Psychoeducation:** You learn about the nature of emotions, how they are experienced, and the impact they have on thoughts, behaviors, and relationships (Fresco et al., 2013).

- **Cognitive restructuring:** You learn to identify and challenge negative or distorted thought patterns that contribute to emotional distress. For example, you may learn to reframe negative self-talk or challenge unrealistic expectations (Stanborough, 2023).

- **Relaxation techniques:** You learn and practice relaxation techniques, such as deep breathing, progressive muscle relaxation, and mindfulness meditation, to calm your nervous system and reduce emotional arousal.

- **Problem-Solving Skills:** You learn to develop effective problem-solving strategies to address challenging situations and manage emotional responses in a more adaptive way.

The benefits: ERTS can help you become more aware of your emotions as they arise, allowing for earlier identification and intervention. You will learn how to manage your emotions more effectively, reducing the frequency and intensity of emotional outbursts. ERTS will also provide you with the right skills to cope with your emotions in a healthy way, which will ultimately lead to improved relationships and reduced anxiety.

How to personalize it: To personalize ERTS, you must first find a qualified therapist. Choose someone you feel comfortable with, as this will be key to the personalization process. You can then work together with your therapist to tailor the ERTS program to your specific needs, allowing you control of the course of action. Further, you can personalize it by choosing which areas of your life you want to incorporate the skills you've acquired through the process.

Physical Activity

What it is: Physical activity refers to any bodily movement that expends energy. This can include a wide range of activities, from moderate-intensity exercise like brisk walking and swimming to more vigorous activities like running, cycling, and team sports.

How it works: Physical activity has a significant impact on the brain and body. When you engage in physical activity, your body releases endorphins, which combat the stress hormone (cortisol). In this way, exercise can help manage your mood and improve your chances of feeling positive. Additionally, physical exercise also increases the levels of neurotransmitters like dopamine and serotonin, which play a major role in regulating mood, motivation, and cognitive function. Regular physical activity can also improve sleep quality, which is essential for emotional well-being and cognitive function.

The benefits: Physical exercise has many benefits. Everyone can benefit from consistent and frequent physical activity, not just ADHDers. However, there are some additional benefits as to why those with ADHD should prioritize exercise not only for physical well-being but because it's good for mental health as well. Here are a few of those benefits to consider:

- reduced stress and anxiety
- improved mood
- increased self-esteem
- improved focus and concentration
- enhanced sleep quality

How to personalize it: Be sure to choose activities that you find enjoyable and motivating. This will increase your likelihood of sticking with them. Begin with short durations and gradually increase the intensity and duration of your workouts as you improve your fitness level. You don't have to exercise at the same time every single day. Switch up when you're being active, as well as what activity you're doing. You might want to go for a walk today, while you might feel like dancing tomorrow. Embrace the flexibility physical exercise offers, and don't put too much pressure on yourself to stick with a specific exercise routine that is rigid. You can also personalize it by choosing to exercise with a friend or on your own, depending on your mood each day.

These tools might feel overwhelming at the moment, or they might not feel precise enough, but it's important to remember that this is not a one-size-fits-all journey. If you feel overwhelmed, slow down and implement one change at a time. These tools are simply the starting blocks. You can take the time to implement these tools in whatever way you want to and then adjust them according to your specific needs. These tools will allow you to build your toolbox of management techniques, providing you with support in every area of your life. In the next chapter, we'll look at some other ways to manage your symptoms, specifically through medicine and treatment.

Chapter 7:

Treatment Options for ADHD

Adults should know that it's never too late to seek help for ADHD. -
Howie Mandel

When it comes to ADHD treatment, opinions are divided, and there are quite a few controversies. While some ADHDers swear by medication and find much relief in using it, others despise it and claim that it "turns them into a zombie." Someone I recently spoke to described taking ADHD medication as "having the ability to turn off the music in my mind." At the end of the day, it remains each ADHDer's choice whether they want to explore ADHD treatment options or not.

No one should pressure you into using medication or seeking treatment if that's not something you're open to. The other tools in this book will serve as a way to help manage your symptoms, allowing you to improve your life without treatment. However, if you are interested in the different treatment options available for ADHD, this is a great place to start that journey. It's good to keep an open mind and make an objective decision. While it might be scary at first, we shouldn't ignore the possible treatment options available. As I like to say, "If you never try, you'll never know."

In this chapter, we'll look at various treatment options, as well as the process of officially obtaining an ADHD diagnosis. The different treatment options include medication, psychological interventions, and lifestyle changes. So, even if you're not open to using medications, be sure to stick around and take a look at the other options, as they might provide you with valuable insight

Understanding the ADHD Diagnosis Process

A diagnosis of ADHD is the first step for many. Unfortunately, it's not a straightforward process. There's no quick test or bloodwork that can show whether you have ADHD or not. It would be amazing if a simple test existed, but that's not how it works. With no clear-cut lab results or an x-ray, ADHD often gets misdiagnosed as something else due to so many overlapping symptoms. When we refer back to Chapter 2, this is especially true in women. Women often get diagnosed with anxiety instead of ADHD, adding to their frustration and struggles.

Many ADHD symptoms are subjective, and not all healthcare professionals take the time and care to help their patients dig deep to find answers. For example, they might ask their patient, "Do you struggle to remember important dates?" To which they might reply, "No." Truth be told, they do struggle to remember important dates, but they have a calendar and three alarms to remind them to check their calendar each day so they don't forget. In other words, they've already adapted their lifestyle and have ways to manage their symptoms, so they don't consider sharing the initial struggle. That's why it's important to work with a healthcare professional who goes above and beyond and who isn't quick to make a diagnosis based on a few subjective questions.

Receiving an official ADHD diagnosis involves a multi-step process that typically includes:

- **Step 1—Self-assessment and consultation:** The first step is to take note of your potential symptoms, such as difficulty focusing, impulsivity, hyperactivity, forgetfulness, and disorganization. Then, take your concerns to your primary care physician and discuss your findings with them. They can rule out any underlying medical conditions and provide a referral to a specialist.

- **Step 2—Comprehensive evaluation:** You'll likely be referred to a mental health professional specializing in ADHD, such as a psychiatrist, psychologist, or pediatrician. The specialist will then conduct a thorough interview to gather information about your symptoms, medical background, family history, developmental milestones, and current functioning. You may also undergo standardized assessments to evaluate attention, impulsivity, and cognitive function.

- **Step 3—Diagnosis and treatment planning:** Based on the evaluation, the specialist will formulate your struggles and determine if you meet the diagnostic criteria for ADHD. In the event you are diagnosed, the specialist will work with you to develop a personalized treatment plan, which may include medication, therapy, and lifestyle changes.

Throughout the process, you should be open and honest with your healthcare provider. It's also okay to seek a second opinion if you don't agree with their opinion and results. While you should remain respectful and kind, you should also advocate for yourself if you feel dismissed or judged. After you have an official diagnosis, you'll be presented with some treatment options. Let's take a closer look at medication as ADHD treatment.

Medication

When someone struggles to see, you don't just tell them to eat more carrots and then send them on their way, right? No. You provide them with options and recommend eyeglasses to help them see better. You might also recommend eating healthier foods to prevent their eyesight from deteriorating even more, but you won't leave it at that. For many ADHDers, medication is like their eyeglasses. But how exactly does it work? ADHD medication increases the levels of neurotransmitters in your brain, specifically boosting your dopamine and norepinephrine to help improve symptoms. The medication basically provides your brain with the neurotransmitters it struggles to produce by itself, allowing you to experience improved attention, reduced hyperactivity, and more managed executive functions (Cleveland Clinic, 2022).

Types of Medication

It might take some trial and error before you find the medication that works best for you. You and your healthcare provider will have to work together to experiment with different kinds of medications based on your unique needs and symptoms, as well as your reaction to the different types of medication. There are various types of medications, including stimulants, non-stimulants, and antidepressants. Here's a quick breakdown of each medication type.

Stimulants

Stimulants are the most common type of ADHD medication (Cleveland Clinic, 2022). They work by increasing the levels of neurotransmitters like dopamine and norepinephrine in your brain, which play an important role in attention and focus. There are two types of stimulants: immediate-release and extended-release. Immediate-release stimulants are normally taken as needed. For example, if you feel like you're drifting off but need to study, you can quickly take one for a boost. However, it can lead to a "crash" after a couple of hours. In general, extended-release medications are taken in the morning, and they can last up to 12 hours. They result in fewer ups and downs but might not have the immediate effect some are looking for. Examples include methylphenidate (like Ritalin LA, Concerta, and Focalin) and amphetamines (like Adderall and Vyvanse).

Non-Stimulants

Non-stimulants work by increasing the norepinephrine in your brain and are less likely to cause addiction. They take much longer to start working than stimulants, so you may only begin to feel their effect after taking the medication for a couple of weeks. However, they can improve your focus and attention for a much longer period of time and won't cause intense ups and downs (Cleveland Clinic, 2022). Common non-stimulant ADHD medications include Strattera, Intuniv, and Kapvay.

Antidepressants

Antidepressants are approved by the FDA for treating ADHD and are often prescribed in combination with a stimulant due to comorbidities. Antidepressants only work on specific neurotransmitters in the brain but not necessarily neurotransmitters affected by ADHD. However, it has been proven effective in treating some of the symptoms of ADHD but not all of them (Cleveland Clinic, 2022).

With all three of these types, there are risks and benefits involved in the process. Risks of these medications include:

- decreased appetite
- irritability
- weight loss
- difficulty sleeping
- anxiety

- minor growth delay

- upset stomach

- change in blood pressure and heart rate

- fatigue

- low or worsening mood

There are also other potential alternatives depending on one's needs, and the above suggestions are only a snapshot. For this reason, it's vital to have open communication with your doctor if you experience any of these side effects and to keep track of your progress.

Psychological Interventions

If you're not interested in medication, there are other ways to better manage your ADHD, one of which is psychological interventions. These are non-medical treatments that focus on developing coping strategies and behavioral techniques to manage symptoms (Tourjman et al., 2022). These interventions can be highly effective in improving attention, organization, and emotional regulation. In other words, the strategies we've discussed specifically in Chapters 5 and 6 will fall within this category of treatment. Here's how this type of treatment can build confidence and help ADHDers focus on their goals (*Psychosocial Treatments*, 2018).

- **Breaking down overwhelm:** ADHD often involves feeling overwhelmed by the sheer volume of tasks. Psychological interventions, such as cognitive-behavioral therapy (CBT), help individuals break down large tasks into smaller, more manageable steps. This "chunking" process reduces anxiety and makes tasks seem less daunting.

- **Prioritization techniques:** These interventions teach individuals how to prioritize tasks effectively. By identifying the most important task and focusing on it first, individuals can avoid getting sidetracked by less important distractions. This single-minded focus improves efficiency and builds confidence as individuals successfully complete prioritized tasks.

- **Developing self-efficacy:** Through successful implementation of learned strategies, individuals with ADHD gain a sense of accomplishment and increased self-efficacy. This boost in confidence motivates them to continue applying these strategies to other areas of their lives.

- **Addressing underlying issues:** Psychological interventions often address underlying issues like low self-esteem, anxiety, and frustration that can arise from ADHD challenges. By addressing these issues, individuals can develop a more positive self-image and approach tasks with greater confidence.

Psychological interventions empower individuals with ADHD to develop the skills and strategies they need to manage their symptoms effectively.

Lifestyle Changes

The last type of treatment you can consider instead of medication and psychological interventions is lifestyle changes. Lifestyle changes mean you intentionally make changes to your current lifestyle to help your mind and body manage your ADHD symptoms more effectively. Lifestyle changes include changes to your sleep schedule, your diet, and how often you exercise. Let's take a closer look at each and how these lifestyle changes can contribute to ADHD management.

Sleep

When ADHDers don't get enough quality sleep, their core symptoms, such as inattention, hyperactivity, and impulsivity, can significantly worsen (Cruz & Nielsen, 2025). During sleep, the brain consolidates memories, restores energy, and regulates various bodily functions. Insufficient sleep disrupts these processes, leading to daytime fatigue, difficulty concentrating, and increased irritability. In individuals with ADHD, these effects can be particularly pronounced as their brains already face challenges with attention and self-regulation. Sleep problems and ADHD often exist in a cyclical relationship (Watson & Cherney, 2020). ADHD symptoms can be worsened by inadequate sleep, which makes it difficult to fall asleep and remain asleep. This can create a vicious cycle that further disrupts sleep patterns and worsens ADHD symptoms over time (Shen et al., 2020).

To ensure that your sleep contributes to ADHD treatment and doesn't worsen it, here are a few things to consider:

- **Establish a consistent sleep schedule:** Maintain a regular sleep-wake cycle, even on weekends, by going to bed and waking up at the same time every day.

- **Create a relaxing bedtime routine:** Wind down an hour or two before bed with a relaxing activity such as a warm bath, reading, or listening to calming music.

- **Optimize your sleep environment:** Ensure a quiet, dark, and cool sleeping environment. Consider using earplugs, an eye mask, or a white noise machine to block out distractions.

- **Limit screen time before bed:** The blue light emitted from electronic devices can interfere with melatonin production, a hormone that regulates sleep. Before going to bed, avoid screens for at least an hour.

- **Regular exercise:** Regular physical activity can improve sleep quality, but avoid strenuous exercise close to bedtime.

- **Limit caffeine and alcohol:** Avoid caffeine and alcohol in the evening, as these substances can interfere with sleep.

- **Address underlying sleep disorders:** If you suspect you have a sleep disorder such as insomnia or sleep apnea, consult with a healthcare professional for evaluation and treatment.

Prioritizing sleep hygiene and addressing any underlying sleep issues will allow you to improve your sleep quality and reduce the severity of your ADHD symptoms.

Exercise

Exercise can impact ADHD symptoms by positively influencing brain chemistry and overall well-being. Physical activity stimulates the release of endorphins, natural mood boosters that can alleviate symptoms of anxiety and depression, which often co-occur with ADHD. Exercise also increases levels of dopamine, a neurotransmitter necessary for attention, focus, and motivation. This dopamine boost can help individuals with ADHD improve their concentration, reduce impulsivity, and enhance their ability to complete tasks (Bryant, 2020). Here are a few recommendations and tips to consider to best support your ADHD with exercise:

- **Find activities you enjoy:** Engage in activities that you find enjoyable and motivating, such as dancing, swimming, hiking, or team sports.

- **Start gradually:** Begin with short durations and gradually increase the intensity and duration of your workouts.

- **Incorporate it into your routine:** Find ways to incorporate physical activity into your daily routine, such as walking during your lunch break, cycling to work, or taking fitness classes in the evening.

- **Find an exercise buddy:** Exercising with a friend or family member can provide motivation and social support.

- **Listen to your body:** Pay attention to your body's signals and rest when you need to. Avoid pushing yourself too hard, especially when starting out.

Diet

Diet can play a significant role in influencing ADHD symptoms. While not a cure, a balanced diet can contribute to improved focus, reduced impulsivity, and better overall well-being (Lange et al., 2023). A balanced diet provides the essential nutrients the brain needs to function optimally. This doesn't mean you have to eat carrot sticks and kale all day, every day. In fact, a balanced meal means adding carbs to your diet more regularly and focusing on proteins and healthy fats. It's also okay to indulge sometimes and have sugar, as long as it's not your norm. Here are a few tips to consider to help with your diet and ADHD management:

- **Limit processed foods:** Processed foods often contain high levels of sugar, unhealthy fats, and artificial additives, which can negatively impact brain function and may exacerbate ADHD symptoms.

- **Reduce sugar intake:** Sugar can cause energy spikes and crashes, making it difficult to concentrate and control impulses.

- **Prioritize whole grains:** Choose whole-grain bread, pasta, and rice over refined grains, which are lower in nutrients and can cause blood sugar spikes.

- **Incorporate healthy fats:** Include sources of healthy fats in your diet, such as nuts, seeds, avocados, and fatty fish like salmon.

- **Stay hydrated:** Dehydration can negatively impact cognitive function, so drink plenty of water throughout the day.

- **Regular mealtimes:** Eating regular meals and snacks throughout the day can help stabilize blood sugar levels and prevent energy crashes.

- **Food journaling:** Keeping a food journal can help you identify any potential dietary triggers for your ADHD symptoms.

It's important to note that the impact of diet on ADHD symptoms can vary significantly from person to person. Consulting with a registered dietitian or a nutritionist can provide personalized guidance and support in developing a healthy and effective dietary plan.

All in all, I hope you feel empowered and equipped to take back some control and make a change in your life. Whether you're on a journey to find natural solutions to manage your symptoms or you're open to exploring the benefits of medications is all up to you. But one thing is true: you don't have to feel hopeless or alone anymore.

Conclusion

Do you remember Megan's story, which I shared with you in the introduction? Well, allow me to share the story of Megan's daughter, Emily, with you.

Emily used to love preschool. Playing with her friends and making up stories was her favorite part of every day. Even during meal times, she made her food talk to one another. But when Emily went to primary school, she showed some signs that felt all too familiar to her mom. She started struggling academically, her friends often misunderstood her, and she was often stuck in her own imaginary world and thoughts and appeared uninterested in what others had to say. Emily's mom brought her to her physician to undergo the whole ADHD diagnostic process, and she was later diagnosed with ADHD-inattentive subtype. Following the diagnosis, Emily received both pharmacological and psychological support. She started to better understand her struggles, and the family implemented support to better support her.

She is currently 15, doing well academically, and establishing good relationships with her peers. Her teachers and parents have seen a significant improvement in how Emily presents herself, as she is more confident and happy than ever. However, Emily's story could've been much different. She could have suffered for half her life the way Megan did. But because of an early diagnosis and the right changes, she is thriving!

Just like Emily, you can also thrive. By using the knowledge and tools provided in this book, you can take back some control and make peace with ADHD. Remember, it's not the enemy. Don't try to fight it—learn how to work with it. I know you are capable of turning these struggles into opportunities to grow and become resilient, finding new ways to manage your ADHD along the way. I trust that you now feel equipped and empowered to make the changes necessary and understand exactly how your mind works.

If this book has helped you in any way, please consider leaving a review so other ADHDers can find their way here as well. I can't wait to hear all your success stories. Now go out there, pass this book on to another ADHDer who needs it, and make the practical changes you need to thrive with your ADHD. You've got this!

References

Adamou, M., Arif, M., Asherson, P., Aw, T.-C., Bolea, B., Coghill, D., Guðjónsson, G., Halmøy, A., Hodgkins, P., Müller, U., Pitts, M., Trakoli, A., Williams, N., & Young, S. (2013). Occupational issues of adults with ADHD. *BMC Psychiatry*, *13*(1). https://doi.org/10.1186/1471-244x-13-59

ADDA Editorial Team. (2023, September 22). A guide for men with ADHD (and their loved ones). https://add.org/adhd-symptoms-in-men/

ADDtitude Editors. (2019, August 30). *What is oppositional defiant disorder (ODD)?* ADDitude. https://www.additudemag.com/what-is-oppositional-defiant-disorder/

ADDitude Editors. (2021, March 24). *ODD vs. ADHD: The facts about oppositional defiant disorder and attention deficit.* ADDitude. https://www.additudemag.com/oppositional-defiant-disorder-odd-and-adhd/

ADDitude Editors, & Perlis, L. B. (2022, May 13). *ADHD, anxiety, and autism: Your AAA guidebook.* ADDitude. https://www.additudemag.com/slideshows/adhd-anxiety-and-autism-symptoms-and-treatment/

ADDitude Editors. (2024, September 30). *17 things to love about ADHD!* ADDitude. https://www.additudemag.com/slideshows/benefits-of-adhd-to-love/

American Psychiatric Association. (2022). *Diagnostic and statistical manual of mental disorders* (5th ed., text rev.). APA Publishing.

Barkley, R. A. (2020). *Taking charge of adult ADHD*. Guilford Press.

Bozhilova, N. S., Michelini, G., Kuntsi, J., & Asherson, P. (2018). Mind wandering perspective on attention-deficit/hyperactivity disorder. *Neuroscience & Biobehavioral Reviews, 92*, 464–476. https://doi.org/10.1016/j.neubiorev.2018.07.010

Brooks, R. (2022, August 9). Quote. In Bader, E. (n.d.). *20+ Best adhd tweets that may confine you to the bed with laughter*. CHEEZburger. https://cheezburger.com/19749125/20-best-adhd-tweets-that-may-confine-you-to-the-bed-with-laughter

Bryant, E. (2020, March 30). *Dopamine affects how brain decides whether a goal is worth the effort*. National Institutes of Health (NIH). https://www.nih.gov/news-events/nih-research-matters/dopamine-affects-how-brain-decides-whether-goal-worth-effort

Burch, K. (2024, July 3). *How to manage sensory overload in ADHD*. Verywell Health. https://www.verywellhealth.com/sensory-overload-and-adhd-5209861

CDC. (2024, May 15). *Data and statistics on ADHD*. https://www.cdc.gov/adhd/data/index.html

Cleveland Clinic. (2022, October 6). *ADHD medications: How they work & side effects*. https://my.clevelandclinic.org/health/treatments/11766-adhd-medication

Cleveland Clinic. (2023a). *Attention deficit disorder (ADHD)*. https://my.clevelandclinic.org/health/diseases/4784-attention-deficithyperactivity-disorder-adhd

Cleveland Clinic. (2023b, January 13) *Depression.* https://my.clevelandclinic.org/health/diseases/9290-depression

Cleveland Clinic. (2024a, March 15). Comorbidities. https://my.clevelandclinic.org/health/articles/comorbidities

Cleveland Clinic. (2024b, March 5). Inattentive ADHD. https://my.clevelandclinic.org/health/diseases/15253-inattentive-adhd

Cornwell, S. (2023, May 2). *Common ADHD myths.* Child Mind Institute. https://childmind.org/article/common-adhd-myths/

Cronkleton, E. (2021, August 13). *What are the differences between and ADHD brain and a neurotypical brain.* Medical News Today. https://www.medicalnewstoday.com/articles/adhd-brain-vs-normal-brain

Cruz, T. R., & Nielsen, J. (2025, January 16). *The connection between sleep and ADHD.* Help Guide. https://www.helpguide.org/wellness/sleep/adhd-and-sleep

Dangmann, C. R., Gunhild K. W. Skogli, Mira, Anne, & Andersen, P. N. (2024). Life gets better: Important resilience factors when growing up with ADHD. *Journal of Attention Disorders, 28*(8), 1198–1209. https://doi.org/10.1177/10870547241246645

DRB. (n.d.). Quote. In ADDitude Editors. (2016, November 28). *10 ADHD quotes to save for a bad day.* ADDitude. https://www.additudemag.com/slideshows/adhd-quotes-for-a-bad-day/

The 5 things proven to motivate ADHD brains. (2024). ADDept. https://www.addept.org/living-with-adult-add-adhd/add-adhd-motivation

Ford, J. D., & Connor, D. F. (2020). ADHD and post-traumatic stress disorder: An examination of shared mechanisms and treatment strategies. *Journal of Clinical Child & Adolescent Psychology, 49*(2), 193-208. https://doi.org/10.1080/15374416.2019.1622123

Fresco, D. M., Mennin, D. S., Heimberg, R. G., & Ritter, M. (2013). Emotion regulation therapy for generalized anxiety disorder. *Cognitive and Behavioral Practice, 20*(3), 282–300. https://doi.org/10.1016/j.cbpra.2013.02.001

Frye, D. (2024, July 29). *What is OCD? Obsessive compulsive disorder explained.* ADDitude. https://www.additudemag.com/what-is-ocd-obsessive-compulsive-disorder/

Green, R. (2023, August 18). *Managing disorganization in ADHD.* Verywell Mind. https://www.verywellmind.com/how-to-recognize-and-manage-disorganization-in-adhd-5216668

Higuera, V. (2019, January 30). *ADHD and ODD: What does it mean if your child has both disorders?* Healthline. https://www.healthline.com/health/adhd/adhd-and-odd#diagnosis

Holmes, G. (2024, May 7). *The untapped strengths of ADHD: Unveiling the hidden gifts.* Enlightened Minds. https://enlightenedminds.co.uk/the-untapped-strengths-of-adhd-unveiling-the-hidden-gifts/

How does ADHD impact problem solving abilities? (2024, June 27). *Focus Bear.* https://www.focusbear.io/blog-post/how-does-adhd-impact-problem-solving-abilities

Hvolby, A. (2014). Associations of sleep disturbance with ADHD: Implications for treatment. *ADHD Attention Deficit and Hyperactivity Disorders*, *7*(1), 1–18. https://doi.org/10.1007/s12402-014-0151-0

James, T. (2024, October 6). *ADHD and note taking: How to feel calm and focused.* Medium. https://medium.com/@theo-james/adhd-and-note-taking-how-to-feel-calm-and-focused-d11ec66f1128

Jordan, A. (2024, October 25). ADHD and its impact on relationships: Understanding challenges. *HealthHero Solutions Limited.* https://www.healthhero.ie/blog/adhd-and-its-impact-on-relationships

Katzman, M. A., Bilkey, T. S., Chokka, P. R., Fallu, A., & Klassen, L. J. (2017). Adult ADHD and comorbid disorders: Clinical implications of a dimensional approach. *BMC Psychiatry*, *17*(1). https://doi.org/10.1186/s12888-017-1463-3

Kelly, K. (n.d.). *ADHD and creativity.* Understood. https://www.understood.org/en/articles/adhd-and-creativity-what-you-need-to-know

Kessler, R. C., Sampson, N. A., Berglund, P., Gruber, M. J., Al-Hamzawi, A., & Andrade, L. (2018). Childhood adversities and adult ADHD: Evidence from the World Mental Health Surveys. *Molecular Psychiatry, 23*(2), 432-441. https://doi.org/10.1038/mp.2017.154

King, P. (2024, August 29). *36 funny quotes about ADHD: Laugh your way through the chaos!* Bonding Health. https://bondinghealth.com/funny-quotes-about-adhd

Kinman, T. (2016, March 22). *Gender differences in ADHD symptoms.* Healthline Media. https://www.healthline.com/health/adhd/adhd-symptoms-in-girls-and-boys#ADHD-and-Gender

Kooij, J. S., Bijlenga, D., Salerno, L., Jaeschke, R., Bitter, I., Balázs, J.,... & Asherson, P. (2019). Updated European Consensus Statement on diagnosis and treatment of adult ADHD. *European Psychiatry, 56,* 14-34. https://doi.org/10.1016/j.eurpsy.2018.11.001

Kranowitz, C. S. (2025, February 14). *3 Types of sensory disorders that look like ADHD.* ADDitude. https://www.additudemag.com/slideshows/signs-of-sensory-processing-disorder/?srsltid=AfmBOoq0EHwV2XuALH64-vq-2rQ20KRjT09Eo6TayMNwPwf_doVez8XM

Lange, K. W., Lange, K., Nakamura, Y., & Reißmann, A. (2023). Nutrition in the management of ADHD: A review of recent research. *Current Nutrition Reports, 12*(3), 383–394. https://doi.org/10.1007/s13668-023-00487-8

Mandel, H. (n.d.). Quote. In ADDitude Editors. (2016, November 28). *10 ADHD quotes to save for a bad day.* ADDitude. https://www.additudemag.com/slideshows/adhd-quotes-for-a-bad-day/

Mayo Clinic Staff. (2022, October 11). *Mindfulness exercises.* Mayo Clinic. https://www.mayoclinic.org/healthy-lifestyle/consumer-health/in-depth/mindfulness-exercises/art-20046356

Mayo Clinic Staff. (2023, December 21). Obsessive-compulsive disorder (OCD). Mayo Clinic. https://www.mayoclinic.org/diseases-conditions/obsessive-compulsive-disorder/symptoms-causes/syc-20354432

Molitor, S. J., Langberg, J. M., & Evans, S. W. (2016). The written expression abilities of adolescents with attention-deficit/hyperactivity disorder. *Research in Developmental*

Disabilities,   *51-52,*   49–59.
https://doi.org/10.1016/j.ridd.2016.01.005

Mooney, J. (n.d.). Quote. In ADDitude Editors. (2016, November 28). *10 ADHD quotes to save for a bad day.* ADDitude. https://www.additudemag.com/slideshows/adhd-quotes-for-a-bad-day/

Morales, T. (2022, September 22). *What is borderline personality disorder? BPD symptoms, treatments & causes.* ADDitude. https://www.additudemag.com/what-is-borderline-personality-disorder-bpd-symptoms/

Morin, A. (n.d.). *8 common myths about ADHD.* Understood. https://www.understood.org/en/articles/common-myths-about-adhd

Mutti-Driscoll, C. J. (2025, January 13). Understanding sustained attention as an executive function. *Psychology Today.* https://www.psychologytoday.com/za/blog/empowerment-is-real/202501/understanding-sustained-attention-as-an-executive-function

Niermann, H. C. M., & Scheres, A. (2014). The relation between procrastination and symptoms of attention-deficit hyperactivity disorder (ADHD) in undergraduate students. *International Journal of Methods in Psychiatric Research,* *23*(4), 411–421. https://doi.org/10.1002/mpr.1440

Normand, S., Schneider, B. H., & Philippe Robaey. (2007). Attention-Deficit/Hyperactivity disorder and the challenges of close friendship. *Journal of the Canadian Academy of Child and Adolescent Psychiatry, 16*(2), 67. https://pmc.ncbi.nlm.nih.gov/articles/PMC2242648/

Novotni, M. (2021, July 8). *Are you listening?* ADDitude. https://www.additudemag.com/adhd-listening-problems/

Novotni, M. (2024, February 28). *ADHD in adults: Problems with eye contact.* ADDitude. https://www.additudemag.com/avoiding-eye-contact/

Olivardia, R. (2021, August 21). *When OCD and ADHD coexist: Symptom presentation, diagnosis, and treatment.* ADDitude. https://www.additudemag.com/ocd-adhd-comorbid-symptoms-diagnosis-treatment/

Ovcharenko, J. (2025, January 6). *ADHD quotes: From sad to inspiring.* Numo ADHD. https://numo.so/journal/adhd-quotes

Pliszka, S. R. (2019). Comorbidity of ADHD and anxiety disorders: Differences in treatment approaches. *Journal of Clinical Psychiatry, 80*(3), 19-24. https://doi.org/10.4088/JCP.18r12473

Psychosocial Treatments. (2018). CHADD. https://chadd.org/for-parents/psychosocial-treatments/

Relationships & social skills. (2018). CHADD. https://chadd.org/for-adults/relationships-social-skills/

Rodden, J. (2019, August 28). *What does oppositional defiant disorder look like in adults?* ADDitude. https://www.additudemag.com/oppositional-defiant-disorder-in-adults/

Rodden, J. (2023, March 28). *What is depression?* ADDitude. https://www.additudemag.com/what-is-depression/

Rodden, J. (2024, July 10). *ASD: What is autism spectrum disorder?* ADDitude. https://www.additudemag.com/what-is-autism-spectrum-disorder-asd/

Roth, E. (2019, April 1). *ADHD and depression: What's the link?* Healthline. https://www.healthline.com/health/adhd/depression#suicidal-thoughts

Seuss. (n.d.). Quote. In McDowell, C.F. (2011, May 20). *Love is weird.* A Reverent Life. https://reverentlife.com/2011/05/30/love-is-weird/

Shen, C., Luo, Q., Chamberlain, S. R., Morgan, S., Romero-Garcia, R., Du, J., Zhao, X., Touchette, É., Montplaisir, J., Vitaro, F., Boivin, M., Tremblay, R. E., Zhao, X.-M., Robaey, P., Feng, J., & Sahakian, B. J. (2020). What is the link between attention-deficit/hyperactivity disorder and sleep disturbance? A Multimodal examination of longitudinal relationships and brain structure using large-scale population-based cohorts. *Biological Psychiatry*, *88*(6), 459–469. https://doi.org/10.1016/j.biopsych.2020.03.010

Sherman, C. (2019, September 26). *Is it ADHD, depression, or both?* ADDitude. https://www.additudemag.com/adhd-and-depression-symptoms-treatment/

Silva, S. (2024, October 10). *What is the role of dopamine in ADHD?* Healthline. https://www.healthline.com/health/adhd/adhd-dopamine

Smith, M. (2025, January 16). Tips for managing adult ADHD. Help Guide. https://www.helpguide.org/mental-health/adhd/managing-adult-adhd

Smith, S. (2025, March 29). *Why ADHD students use humor to mask.* Medium. https://medium.com/@sol_smith/why-adhd-students-use-humor-to-mask-7c5390cbc6fa

Smith-Ruetz, J. (n.d.). Quote. In Dahl, D. (2023, April 8). *80 Adhd quotes about the neurodivergent way of paying attention.* Everyday Power. https://everydaypower.com/adhd-quotes/

Staley, B. S., Robinson, L. R., Claussen, A. H., Katz, S. M., Danielson, M. L., Summers, A. D., Farr, S. L., Blumberg, S. J., & Tinker, S. C. (2024). Attention-Deficit/Hyperactivity disorder diagnosis, treatment, and telehealth use in adults — national center for health statistics rapid surveys system, united states, october–november 2023. *MMWR. Morbidity and Mortality Weekly Report, 73*(40), 890–895. https://doi.org/10.15585/mmwr.mm7340a1

Stanborough, R. J. (2023, June 5). *How to change negative thinking with cognitive restructuring.* Healthline. https://www.healthline.com/health/cognitive-restructuring

Sullivan, R. M., Riccio, D. C., & González, A. (2019). ADHD, trauma, and risk-taking behaviors: A developmental perspective. *Development and Psychopathology, 31*(4), 1167-1180. https://doi.org/10.1017/S0954579419000679

Think ADHD. (2024, September 25). *ADHD and hyperfocus.* Think ADHD. https://thinkadhd.co.uk/adhd-and/adhd-and-hyperfocus/

Tourjman, V., Louis-Nascan, G., Ahmed, G., DuBow, A., Côté, H., Daly, N., Daoud, G., Espinet, S., Flood, J., Gagnier-Marandola, E., Gignac, M., Graziosi, G., Mansuri, Z., & Sadek, J. (2022). Psychosocial interventions for attention deficit/hyperactivity disorder: A systematic review and meta-analysis by the CADDRA guidelines work GROUP. *Brain Sciences*, *12*(8), 1023. https://doi.org/10.3390/brainsci12081023

Vanicek, T., Spies, M., Rami-Mark, C., Savli, M., Höflich, A., Kranz, G. S., Hahn, A., Kutzelnigg, A., Traub-Weidinger, T., Mitterhauser, M., Wadsak, W., Hacker, M., Volkow, N. D., Kasper, S., & Lanzenberger, R. (2014). The norepinephrine transporter in attention-deficit/hyperactivity disorder investigated with positron emission tomography. *JAMA Psychiatry*, *71*(12), 1340. https://doi.org/10.1001/jamapsychiatry.2014.1226

Volkow, N. D., Wang, G. J., Newcorn, J., Kollins, S. H., Wigal, T. L., & Telang, F. (2021). Brain circuits involved in ADHD and anxiety: Overlapping mechanisms. *Nature Reviews Neuroscience*, *22*(7), 439-453. https://doi.org/10.1038/s41583-021-00450-w

Watson, S. (2024, May 27). *ADHD and substance abuse.* WebMD. https://www.webmd.com/add-adhd/adhd-and-substance-abuse-is-there-a-link

Watson, S., & Cherney, K. (2020, May 15). *Sleep deprived? Here is what lack of sleep does to your body.* Healthline. https://www.healthline.com/health/sleep-deprivation/effects-on-body#effects

Weiss, M., Murray, C., & Weiss, G. (2020). The impact of PTSD on individuals with ADHD: Clinical challenges and treatment considerations. *Journal of Attention Disorders*, *24*(12), 1757-1766. https://doi.org/10.1177/1087054719878162

Wilens, T. E., Biederman, J., Faraone, S. V., Martelon, M., Westerberg, D., & Spencer, T. J. (2009). Presenting ADHD symptoms, subtypes, and comorbid disorders in clinically referred adults with ADHD. *The Journal of*

Clinical Psychiatry, *70*(11), 1557–1562. https://doi.org/10.4088/jcp.08m04785pur

Wilkins, F. (2024, April 10). *How is the ADHD brain different?* Child Mind Institute. https://childmind.org/article/how-is-the-adhd-brain-different/

www.ingramcontent.com/pod-product-compliance
Lightning Source LLC
Chambersburg PA
CBHW051246020426
42333CB00025B/3084